THE PICTURE

IMAGES OF MEDICINE AND PHARMACY

OF HEALTH

This exhibition and catalogue are made possible by a grant from Merck & Co., Inc., in honor of its Centennial.

Philadelphia Museum of Art

THE PICTURE

IMAGES OF MEDICINE AND PHARMACY

OF HEALTH

From the William H. Helfand Collection

Commentaries by William H. Helfand

Essays by Patricia Eckert Boyer, Judith Wechsler, and Maurice Rickards

Distributed by the University of Pennsylvania Press

Sponsor's Statement

Today's health care system is a complex mix of professionals and patients, medical ideas and values, technologies and treatments, as well as public and private institutions ranging from the neighborhood doctor's office to government agencies and multinational pharmaceutical firms like Merck. As participants in this system, we all have a vital stake in understanding its policies, paradoxes, and promises. But the complexity of modern medicine can be daunting. How can we meet the challenge of improving public awareness of the nature of modern health care?

This exhibition provides an intriguing answer. This selection of medical and pharmaceutical prints, posters, and caricatures from the William H. Helfand Collection both educates and entertains. A pharmacist and chemical engineer by training, Bill Helfand was a long-time Merck executive. His perceptive eye targeted images that illustrate how views of doctors and pharmacists, and health care in general, have shifted over the past two hundred years. The essays in this catalogue add interesting perspectives to help us interpret the signs and symbols on display.

The Picture of Health is thus a mirror reflecting the changing historical relationships of medicine and society. As we celebrate the values and vision that have shaped Merck's first century, it is our pleasure to join with the Philadelphia Museum of Art in sponsoring this provocative exhibition on aspects of pharmacy and medicine in modern culture.

Roy Vagelos

P. Roy Vagelos, M.D.
Chairman and Chief Executive Officer
Merck & Co., Inc.

Contents

Foreword

What do a curvaceously exuberant poster by Jules Chéret, a sprightly trade card extolling the virtues of Bright's Kidney Beans, and a merciless caricature of King Louis-Philippe of France by Honoré Daumier have in common? Their mutual origin in the imaginative and provocative interaction between the visual arts and the history of medicine and pharmacy, and the fascination they hold for a passionate collector deeply interested in both fields. For nearly twenty-five years the Department of Prints, Drawings, and Photographs at the Philadelphia Museum of Art has been the beneficiary of the generosity, expertise, and energetic support of William H. Helfand, and this exhibition is the delightful result.

In 1967, having assembled a collection of over four hundred prints and printed materials with medical subjects, Bill Helfand's interest was drawn to the Museum's Ars Medica collection, which had been shaped first by Carl Zigrosser as Curator of Prints and then by his successor Kneeland McNulty. Ars Medica, a term invented for the Museum's holdings by the erudite and resourceful Zigrosser, was encouraged by a sequence of major grants from SmithKline Beecham over many decades and now encompasses a wealth of works of art and images from Europe and the United States over seven centuries, ranging from the magisterial, anatomical woodcuts of Vesalius to Robert Rauschenberg's huge silkscreen based on an X ray of his own body. Bill Helfand's enthusiasm for the Museum's collection, which numbers over 1,500 works, quickly developed into a working relationship with the Department that has continued to the present day. Throughout Bill's career as an executive with Merck Sharp & Dohme in Philadelphia, Paris, and New York, and since his retirement, he has continued not only to add to his own collection (which now includes over 25,000 items), but he has also pursued and donated works to the Museum, participated in exhibitions and publications of the Ars Medica collection, and worked countless hours on identifying and classifying our prints and drawings with medical subjects. In 1986, Bill made the magnificent offer to donate over a period of years any works from his collection selected by the Museum. From his first two large gifts that followed in 1988 and 1989, most of the present exhibition has been selected.

Three specialists on the subjects of printed posters, caricatures, and ephemera have contributed thoughtful essays to the catalogue that put each group of objects in context, and for that we are grateful to Patricia Eckert Boyer, Judith Wechsler, and Maurice Rickards. The catalogue entries have been written, most appropriately, by Bill Helfand, who has been deeply involved with research and publication on the objects in his collection for so many years. The publication of the catalogue was overseen with characteristic zeal by George H. Marcus, while Sherry Babbitt as Editor gave the text her customary enthusiastic and thorough attention; Phillip Unetic conceived the catalogue's design, which so efficiently captures the liveliness of the material therein.

Ellen S. Jacobowitz, during her tenure as Research Curator for Prints at the Museum, worked with Bill Helfand to arrive at the initial selection of the exhibition. The staff of the Conservation Center for Art and Historic Artifacts in Philadelphia, particularly its Chief Conservator Glen Ruzicka and Senior Conservator Nancy Ash, gave much time and expertise to the treatment of many of the objects, as did Faith H. Zieske, the Museum's Associate Conservator of Works of Art on Paper. Phoebe Toland and Gary Hiatt advised on the presentation and installation of the works, and Graydon Wood and Andrew Harkins spent many hours on the photography of the objects for the catalogue. In the Department of Prints, Drawings, and Photographs, Starr Figura, Curatorial Intern, helped with cataloguing and organizing the objects, and Rhonda V. Davis, Departmental Secretary, coped with the details of keeping the exhibition lists and photographs in order.

With the encouragement of Bill Helfand, The Merck Company Foundation was approached for support of the exhibition. We were delighted by the enthusiastic response to the collection by the staff of The Merck Company Foundation and overjoyed by their agreement to fund all aspects of the exhibition and its catalogue in honor of the one-hundredth anniversary of Merck & Co., Inc. We are deeply grateful to P. Roy Vagelos, M.D., Chairman and Chief Executive Officer of Merck & Co., Inc., and Albert D. Angel, Vice President, Public Affairs, as well as to Charles R. Hogen, Jr., Executive Vice President, The Merck Company Foundation. Dr. Jeffrey L. Sturchio, Corporate Archivist, has been the helpful and knowledgeable coordinator of contact between the Museum and The Merck Company Foundation.

We join with Bill Helfand and our colleagues at Merck & Co., Inc., in the hope that this lively array of images, assembled with so much care for the light that they shed not only upon the annals of medicine but on the history of taste, style, and political vicissitudes as well, will reach a large and interested public through this exhibition, even as they will enrich the Museum's permanent collection for generations to come.

Anne d'Harnoncourt
The George D. Widener Director

Innis Howe Shoemaker
Senior Curator of Prints, Drawings, and Photographs

Preface

I acquired my first prints from Berthe von Moschzisker of The Print Club of Philadelphia in the early 1950s. These works by Francisco Goya, Georges Rouault, and Giovanni Battista Piranesi are still on my walls, and still provide me with a great deal of pleasure. But shortly after I made these early purchases, I received a catalogue from the British book dealers Elkin Mathews listing a 1772 caricature, *The Chymical Macaroni, Capn Ludgate*, that I was able to acquire. The captain was only slightly caricatured; he was holding a mortar and pestle labeled "Cantharides," and inscribed on the oddly shaped queue on his wig was "Family Medicine Chests neatly fitted up." At the time I was beginning my career in the pharmaceutical industry, and the image of a man holding an identifiable pharmaceutical symbol seemed relevant. I wondered if other prints on medical themes existed and thus began a lengthy quest that still continues.

I discovered quickly that there are indeed many prints relating to medical, pharmaceutical, and dental subjects, including portraits, caricatures, posters, and *imagerie populaire*, or popular prints. There are also a wide variety of advertisements and other printed ephemera that fall into this broad category of medical images. At the same time I discovered like-minded collectors, several of whom were willing to give advice to a neophyte. With many questions and problems in mind, and with some trepidation, I called on Kneeland McNulty, then Curator of Prints, Drawings, and Photographs at the Philadelphia Museum of Art, and soon found a receptive audience for my concerns as well as a knowledgeable mentor. I also learned that in the late 1940s, through the generosity of Smith, Kline & French (now SmithKline Beecham), the Museum had established a fund for the acquisition of works of art on paper related to medicine. In 1952 the Department had first assembled and exhibited a group of these medical prints as the "Ars Medica Collection."

Thus began my long and fruitful association with the Philadelphia Museum of Art. Working with Kneeland McNulty, I assisted in the growth of the Ars Medica holdings, and after his retirement participated in its further development with Ellen S. Jacobowitz, Diane R. Karp, and most recently Innis Howe Shoemaker, who has carried this project, the most recent in a series of exhibitions and publications devoted to the subject of Ars Medica, to fruition. While there are other active collections of medical prints, the Ars Medica collection of the Philadelphia Museum of Art is distinguished by being the only one housed in an art museum, all of the others being subdivisions of medical libraries.

My own collection of medical and pharmaceutical prints grew too, particularly during the years my family and I lived abroad. However, as the years have gone by, I have found my interests moving more and more toward the popular arts. Having spent a large part of my career in pharmaceutical marketing with Merck & Co., I was attracted to prints with a message, objects whose intent was not just to create an attractive image but also to influence the viewer. The posters and printed advertisements that captured my attention clearly had a purpose, as did the caricatures, especially those created in response to political events. Even certain printed ephemera, song sheets, and comic valentines, for example, fall into the category of such popular prints. I found that most of the objects of importance to me incorporated text with the images in order to communicate more forcefully. What I have always considered essential, however, was to find a work of art that balanced artistic merit with social purpose.

The objects chosen for *The Picture of Health* have been assembled from three of the major areas that have been of particular interest to me: posters, caricatures, and printed ephemera. The exhibition includes works by several artists who were major contributors to the popular arts, including Leonetto Cappiello, Jules Chéret, Alfred Concanen, Adolphe-Louis-Charles Crespin, George Cruikshank, Honoré Daumier, Adolf Hohenstein, André Gill, James Gillray, Thomas Rowlandson, and Théophile-Alexandre Steinlen. The Museum's Ars Medica collection, rich as it is with superb prints, drawings, and photographs, is further enhanced by the addition of such examples. Thus these objects should reinforce and expand the significance of the Museum's collection and make it more valuable to those who will use it.

While many of the objects in this selection depict medical scenes or comment on health images, I would be the first to admit that occasionally the medical aspect is only marginal, but it has been a necessary condition for me to acquire these works. Without some organizing principle, such as the one that has been my long-lasting concern, the size of the collection might otherwise have been overwhelming. Over the years, many people have played an active part in building my collection, and it is not possible to list all of the collectors, dealers, curators, and librarians who have helped. But I must single out my deep gratitude to my wife, Audrey, who has contributed to its development in a thousand ways and who has continued to do so in creating this exhibition. Also through the years, my collection has brought me enormous pleasure, has served as my source for a number of publications and exhibitions on medical and pharmaceutical subjects, and has proved useful to other scholars and researchers. I have always wanted it to be used as much as possible; there is no better way to accomplish this goal than to make it part of the Ars Medica collection of the Philadelphia Museum of Art.

William H. Helfand

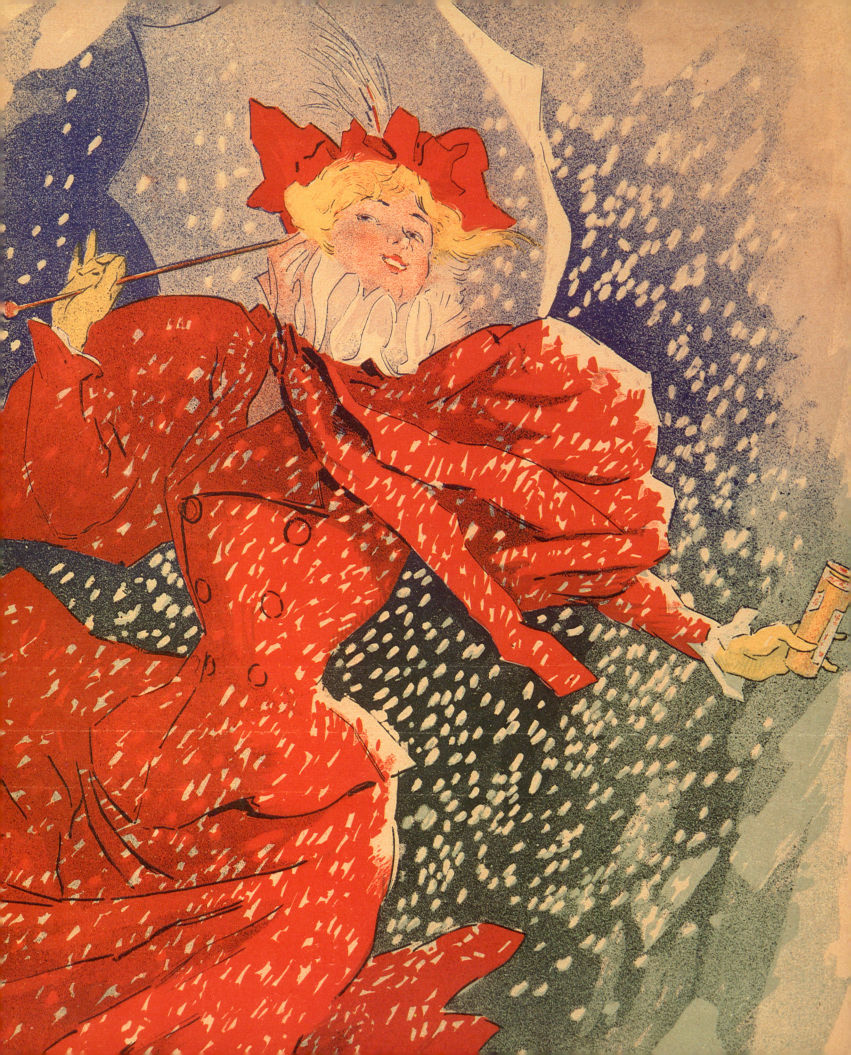

To Delight and Provoke: The Poster in the Service of Medicine

Patricia Eckert Boyer

As a means of communication, the poster has a dual role: it must both sell a product or an idea and captivate and convince through the use of image and a minimal amount of type. When most successful, the poster is also an art form. It was in the latter part of the nineteenth century, first in France and shortly thereafter in other countries, that posters came to be appreciated for their artistic potential as well as for their commercial possibilities. From that moment on, those who commissioned these works became the patrons of a large group of artists who struggled to attain a balance between art and message that assured the vitality and success of their medium. Manufacturers of health care products and government agencies promoting public health quickly identified the large, illustrated poster as a powerful vehicle for the broad dissemination of information, and put it into service in achieving their objectives.

The history of public announcements can be traced back to antiquity. But the earliest printed advertisement to appear in England was made in 1477, and in France one of the first illustrated placards promoted umbrellas in 1715.[1] However, prior to the nineteenth century, public announcements, or posters, pasted on walls or hoardings were small and usually consisted primarily of typography, with little or no illustration or other decorative embellishment.[2] They were printed as inexpensive multiples through the process of either wood or copper engraving. Both of these techniques limited the size of the poster to the dimensions of either the block of wood or the plate of copper. The physical challenges of incising into these surfaces also restricted the size of the printed placard.

Gradually, however, with the invention of lithography in the mid-1790s by the German Aloys Senefelder, the poster began to change. Because of the simplicity of the lithographic process in which artists could draw directly onto the stone, lithography was soon explored as a medium for original expression.

1. See John Barnicoat, *A Concise History of Posters: 1870—1970* (New York, 1972), p. 8.

2. Among the few exceptions to this were military recruiting posters and some woodcut posters. See Dawn Ades et al., *Posters: The Twentieth-Century Poster—Design of the Avant-Garde* (New York, 1984), p. 25.

Théodore Géricault, Francisco Goya, and Eugène Delacroix were among the first prominent artists to devote significant attention to the process. Despite such early artistic successes, however, by the middle of the nineteenth century lithography was used mostly as an inexpensive reproductive medium. Illustrated lithographic posters first appeared in France in the 1830s, when publishers began to advertise new books with black-and-white posters drawn by their illustrators.[3]

One man, Jules Chéret, was responsible for resurrecting artistic lithography and adapting the poster to the possibilities afforded by the relatively new process of color lithography. Beginning in the 1860s, he created large, colorful images that were used for advertising, and in doing so he elevated the commercial placard to the rank of art.[4] Chéret introduced a system of color printing in which a different lithographic stone carries each of the colors used in the finished work. When superimposed, they created full-color compositions such as his posters for Vin Mariani (no. 7) and Pastilles Géraudel (no. 8). By dividing his image among the various stones, each carrying a portion of the design, Chéret was also able to increase the size of his posters. His great success established the poster as a means of artistic expression and encouraged an entire generation to follow his lead, thereby initiating what has come to be called the golden age of poster making.

Chéret's redefinition of the poster as a powerful artistic medium also responded to the transformation of Paris that had occurred during the Second Empire (1852–70), when Georges Eugène Haussmann replaced large sections of the city's narrow, winding medieval streets with a network of grand boulevards lined with monumental buildings.[5] The new expanses of neutral wall encouraged the pasting of placards, while the broad new avenues dictated that these posters should become larger and bolder in order to be legible and attractive at greater distances. Chéret's posters were the first to bring art to the streets, making it accessible to everyone. The critic Roger Marx, recognizing Chéret's contribution, wrote in 1889 that

Chéret's task was to rescue the drab streets from the monotony of the perfectly straight rows of houses and fill them with the fireworks of color, the animation of movement, and the radiance of joy; to convert the foundations into surfaces to be decorated and to compel this open-air museum to reflect the character of the nation and to promote the unconscious training of taste. A thousand magical and laughing visions, masked as advertisements, sprang from the impulses of his genius. He elevated the poster to the status of the mural.[6]

Chéret designed more than a thousand posters, twenty-one of which were for medical and pharmaceutical products. His innovative approach to this graphic medium inspired numerous artists, including Pierre Bonnard, Henri de Toulouse-Lautrec, Théophile-Alexandre Steinlen (see no. 22), and Eugène Grasset, who were intrigued by the formal and technical possibilities of color lithography. Manufacturers of medical products, publishers, dance-hall own-

3. A. Hyatt Mayor, *Prints & People: A Social History of Printed Pictures* (New York, 1971), fig. 640.

4. See Camille Mauclair, *Jules Chéret* (Paris, 1930).

5. See David H. Pinkney, *Napoleon III and the Rebuilding of Paris* (Princeton, 1958).

6. Roger Marx, "Jules Chéret," preface for La Bodinière, Paris, *Catalogue de l'exposition des oeuvres de Jules Chéret* (December 1889); reprinted in Roger Marx, *L'Art social* (Paris, 1913), pp. 154–55.

ers—indeed anyone with an idea or good to promote—would learn to take advantage of its commercial and creative potential.

This intense artistic activity soon gave rise to an equally strong interest in posters among collectors. By the early 1890s posters were often stripped from the walls by eager collectors, even before the paste had dried. In 1891 the Parisian art dealer Edmond Sagot published an illustrated catalogue of over one hundred pages, listing some 2,200 posters that he offered for sale.[7] Two years later Charles Hiatt, an English collector who was quick to appreciate French posters, expressed his enthusiasm by suggesting that "the print collector, wearied for the moment of engravings or etchings, might, without loss of dignity, turn his attention to the wall-pictures that gaily decorate the tedious new streets of Paris."[8]

Although the bold, colorful compositions of Chéret and Toulouse-Lautrec are today seen as representative of the period, in fact the French poster movement of the 1890s embraced a range of styles. In the color lithograph *Office Médical* (no. 11), for example, lingering strains of classicism are evident in the design, which is sedate in comparison to Chéret's rococo frivolity. In another example, the designer of the poster advertising the Fête Parisienne to aid cholera victims (no. 5) chose to avoid the use of color and instead exploited the somber tonal possibilities of the lithograph, which he may have felt conveyed an atmosphere more appropriate to the cause he was promoting.

In general the styles of the late nineteenth century prevailed in the French posters of the early twentieth century as well. The Symbolism of Lucien Lévy-Dhurmer, one of the movement's greatest proponents, is apparent in his poster for a benefit for soldiers infected with tuberculosis (no. 25). The gritty style of the caricatures seen in much of Steinlen's work of the 1890s likewise reappears in a more realistic and descriptive incarnation in his *Soldier, the Country Relies on You* of 1916 (no. 22).

The only artist working in France to devise a new aesthetic spirit for the twentieth-century poster was the Italian-born Leonetto Cappiello, who arrived in Paris in 1898 at the age of twenty-three. His stylistic innovation of associating a figure with the product and making that figure spring forth from a neutral background—"the science of the blot," as he called it—was intended to capture the attention of the passerby.[9] The powerful effect of this device is apparent in his *Katabexine* of 1903 (no. 17), where the depiction of the woman is very much rooted in nineteenth-century conventions, but the use of the dark background from which the figure readily stands out demonstrates Cappiello's contribution to the art of the poster. In his *Le Thermogène* of 1909 (no. 18), a fire-breathing circus performer personifies the advertised product: wads of cotton permeated with a chemical that creates the sensation of heat. With this poster Cappiello had expressed both his own mature style and the formula for the twentieth-century poster. His influence was tremendous, and many artists, including Michel Liébeaux (see no. 28), imitated his style.

7. Edmond Sagot, *Catalogue d'affiches illustrées, anciennes et modernes* (Paris, 1891).

8. Charles T. J. Hiatt, "The Collecting of Posters: A New Field for Connoisseurs," *The Studio*, vol. 1 (May 1893), p. 61.

9. Alain Weill, *The Poster: A Worldwide Survey and History* (Boston, 1985), p. 126.

Interest in the art poster spread rapidly outside of France, first to Belgium, where there was already a strong commitment to the applied arts. Adolphe-Louis-Charles Crespin designed some of the finest Belgian posters of the late nineteenth century. His *Love Conquers All* (no. 9), for example, displays his bold and almost architectonic sense of design and ornamentation. In America, Will Bradley, Louis Rhead, and Edward Penfield were among the important poster artists. The well-known illustrator Maxfield Parrish also designed several posters, and early in his career won a poster competition in a field that included over six hundred entries.[10] Parrish's *No-To-Bac* (no. 4) exemplifies his emerging detailed, narrative style. Among the Spanish artists to respond to the growing interest in the poster was Ramón Casas, who had lived in Paris, where he was perhaps most influenced by poster artists such as Steinlen (see no. 22) and Henri-Gabriel Ibels (see no. 71), who depicted society's victims as well as its stars. This is certainly apparent in Casas's *Syphilis* (no. 12), where the female figure recalls Steinlen's images of working women.

Adolf Hohenstein was arguably the most important poster designer in Italy at the turn of the century. Although of German origin, he lived and worked in Milan, where he directed the art department of the Ricordi printing firm. Hohenstein's compositional solution departed dramatically from the French conventions that were so often emulated in other posters of the period. With its combination of photographically realistic figures with vivid colors and a melodramatic play of light and shade, the image he created for the 1900 hygiene exhibition in Naples (no. 14) is typical of his novel approach to the poster. Here he presents a heroic family drinking from a clean mountain stream—the fountain of life—that is the source of the light, air, water, and exercise that are the keys to their good health. The figures emerge from their spacious vignette and through the linear, undulating frame and colorful barrier that separate their idealized, mythical world from the reality of the viewer.

The poster did not flourish in late nineteenth-century Germany as it did in most of Europe and America. As Julius Meier-Graefe wrote in 1896, "it is difficult to speak of the German poster because properly speaking, the poster as conceived in France does not exist . . . . Advertising in big cities makes use almost exclusively of newspapers."[11] Fernand Schultz-Wettel's 1902 poster for the bandage manufacturer C. Degen & Cie (no. 16) does exemplify the academic realism that dominated many early German posters. On the other hand, Carl Kunst's *Dr. Dessauer's Touring Apotheke* (no. 20) is a bold composition of highly stylized forms and patches of flat color that reflects the formidable development of the German poster that had occurred by about 1910. Kunst's image contains traces of the Jugendstil, the German counterpart of French Art Nouveau, in the outlining of natural forms and letters. It also incorporates elements of the *Sach Plakat*, or "object poster," a concept developed around 1906 by the artist Lucian Bernhard, whose reductive formula was to show only the image of the product and the name of the manufacturer, and to incorporate strong coloring and compelling typography

10. Ibid., p. 79.

11. Quoted in ibid., p. 95.

into highly stylized compositions.[12] Kunst, however, retained a narrative context for the product his poster promoted.

L ithography was introduced into Japan in the late 1870s, and the first lithographic poster was printed there in the early 1890s. But it was not until the Russo-Japanese War ended in 1905 that the Japanese devoted any real effort to advertising and thus to posters. Although Western poster artists of the late nineteenth century were profoundly inspired by the strong colors, vigorously juxtaposed patterns, and elevated asymmetry of Japanese woodblock prints,[13] the Japanese did not find the same bold and successful applications for their native artistic formulas. For example, the designer of *Iyanaga Eye Medicine* (no. 2) largely ignored the powerful potential of the image to attract buyers for the advertised product and disseminate information to a large audience. Instead the figures are restricted to the corner of the composition, leaving the lengthy text to sell the product.

While the power of the poster to dispense information to the public was well recognized by private business before the end of the nineteenth century, governments had not officially used this art form until World War I, when the need to recruit soldiers spurred governmental patronage of poster artists. Perhaps the most famous American example is James Montgomery Flagg's figure of Uncle Sam pointing to the viewer and saying, "I want YOU for the U.S. Army."[14] Others were concerned with the soldiers' health and welfare. Steinlen's *Soldier, the Country Relies on You* (no. 22), for example, warns servicemen of the perils of syphilis. Posters were also used to raise money for various war-related causes. Lévy-Dhurmer designed an image to promote a national fundraiser for soldiers with tuberculosis (no. 25).

It is not surprising that posters, with their ability to capture the interest of large numbers of people, have often been used to address issues of public health.[15] In Casas's 1895 advertisement for a sanatorium for syphilitics, the afflicted woman (almost certainly a prostitute) grasps behind her the serpent that symbolizes the evil—sexual promiscuity—that has resulted in her infection, and looks longingly at the white lily, a symbol of her lost purity and by extension of her former good health. The snake, traditionally a generic symbol for evil, became a very popular *fin-de-siècle* motif. Its impact continues, and received a modern application in David Lance Goines's *AIDS Prevention* of 1985 (no. 31). Furthermore, just as early posters were used to publicize the Fête Parisienne for the benefit of cholera victims (no. 5) and to call for donations for the Italian Red Cross (no. 26), in 1985 Paul Davis created a powerful image to promote an event organized to help people with AIDS (no. 32).

Artists have used a wide variety of means to put forth the items or concepts illustrated in their posters. Some have advertised a product with a theatrical gesture of presentation, as in *Pastilles Valda* of about 1930 (no. 29), where the gentleman aggressively encourages the viewer to use these cough drops. Dressed in a tuxedo and fashionable spectacles, he seems to be both a professional and a dandy, which makes his endorsement of the product author-

12. Ibid., p. 100.

13. See Gabriel P. Weisberg et al., *Japonisme: Japanese Influence on French Art, 1854–1901* (Cleveland, 1975).

14. Stuart Wrede, *The Modern Poster* (New York, 1988), p. 20, fig. 10.

15. See William H. Helfand, "Art in the Service of Public Health: The Illustrated Poster," *Caduceus*, vol. 6, no. 2 (Summer 1990), pp. 1–37.

itative as well as *au courant*. In contrast, Ayer's Sarsaparilla was offered by an avuncular advocate in an American poster of the 1890s (no. 10). Both examples exemplify the rather vernacular, narrative type of placard that co-existed with those of a more contemporary design. Other artists, including Chéret, adopted a more unspecific and universal approach to making the image arresting and the product appealing. Whether advertising lozenges (no. 8), tonic wine (no. 7), or the Moulin Rouge nightclub,[16] the message of Chéret's posters was the same: "Take this, and be delighted!" By contrast Cappiello's great contribution to the success of the illustrated poster—the juxtaposition of a figure that personified the product with a stark background—created an element of surprise that imprinted the image on the mind of the viewer.

Others have used conflict to convey their messages, a technique that has been particularly effective in the posters admonishing the public to avoid certain diseases. In his poster warning soldiers of the dangers of venereal disease (no. 22), Steinlen made the rather crudely didactic contrast between the amorous tart embracing a soldier and the forlorn syphilitic outside the hospital. At the top, a handsome, healthy soldier is framed by flags and laurel boughs, while a skull and crossbones appears among withering vines below. The message could not have been clearer nor more direct.

Similarly direct in its presentation of the ghastly consequences of illicit activities is the 1930s poster advertising the motion picture *Marihuana: Weed with Roots in Hell* (no. 30). Just as Steinlen depicted the battle between good and evil, health and disease, the artist has here extremely effectively conveyed the tension created by the feelings of attraction and repulsion that are aroused simultaneously by this drug that produces both "unleashed passions" and "misery."

Conflict is also the theme in T. Corbella's poster promoting the fight against tuberculosis (no. 27), for the skeletal personification of the disease holds a weapon that has been broken by the onslaught of good hygiene, sunshine, fresh air, rest, temperance, and healthy food. In *A Great Scourge: Tuberculosis* of about 1920 by F. Galais (no. 24), the struggle presented seems to be not only between human beings and the disease but also between the wealthy and the poor, for the artist has set his dismal scene in a poor urban neighborhood in which children and animals rummage through household garbage discarded in the gutters, and women lean out of windows to dump refuse directly onto passersby. By dramatic contrast, in his poster for the 1900 hygiene exhibition Hohenstein uses an idealized setting to emphasize the elements of good health (no. 14). Despite its mythic dimensions, the almost photorealistic depiction of the family makes their state of purity appear somehow more attainable, as though through the practice of good hygiene alone viewers can achieve a life like theirs.

Posters for events held to raise money for the victims of disease often use pathos to convey their message. The French poster announcing the Parisian benefit for those suffering from cholera presents a vignette of a dying child held by his mother within the pyramidal composition of a Pietà (see no. 5). Lévy-Dhurmer's poster promoting the fundraiser for French servicemen with tuberculosis is likewise an almost spiritual image (no. 25). The rather pathetic older man stands silhouetted against a blossoming tree and looks toward a sunlit coastal city, possibly one in which he can take a cure.

In his tremendously poignant contemporary poster for an AIDS benefit, Paul Davis has cast his protagonist, like Lévy-Dhurmer's aging soldier, as a pathetic outsider (no. 32). The singer evokes the tragic clown in the opera *Pagliacci*, one who is meant to bring laughter to others but who is himself dying of a broken heart. Davis may also have chosen a theatrical figure for his image to call attention to the fact that the entertainment industry has been especially affected by the AIDS epidemic.

With the rise of radio and television advertisements as well as the advances in photographic printing technologies, the illustrated poster no longer holds the status it once did. Yet as these examples of images in the service of medicine and pharmacy have shown, the poster has long been a rich source of artistic challenge and variety. Furthermore, the work of Paul Davis and his contemporaries effectively demonstrates that the poster is quite able to maintain its vitality and originality as both an art form and a means of communication.

1

The Celebrated Oxygenated Bitters
Anonymous, American
1846–47
Color woodcut and relief print
23⁷⁄₈ x 18⁵⁄₈″ (60.6 x 47.3 cm)
1991-24-4

Bitters are drinks, usually alcoholic, containing gentian, quinine, quassia, or other bitter-tasting vegetable drugs, that over the years have been recommended for almost every human ill. The Celebrated Oxygenated Bitters, one of a small group that did not contain alcohol, were promoted for dyspepsia, asthma, and general debility, conditions that would seem to have little in common. In this poster of 1846–47, one of the earliest multicolor woodcuts published in the United States, a portrait of the company's proprietor, George B. Green, is prominently illustrated, surrounded by testimonials from five senators, four congressmen, the president of the Michigan State Bank, and "other prominent Gentlemen."

2

Iyanaga Eye Medicine
Anonymous, Japanese
c. 1850–60
Color woodcut
14¹⁄₄ x 19³⁄₁₆″ (36.2 x 48.7 cm)
1981-114-22

Iyanaga was one of many Japanese "patent" medicines, which were usually dispensed by physicians in their offices. In contrast to Western advertising posters, which generally employ large images and little text, most of this example is taken up with text, with only a small illustration of a physician and his aide administering the eye medicine to their patient in the lower right. The calligraphy describes the history and merits of the product, which was manufactured by the Kuno family of Akizuki Yanaga in Chikuzen (now Fukuoka) Province, the ophthalmic problems it was meant to treat, and the directions for its use.

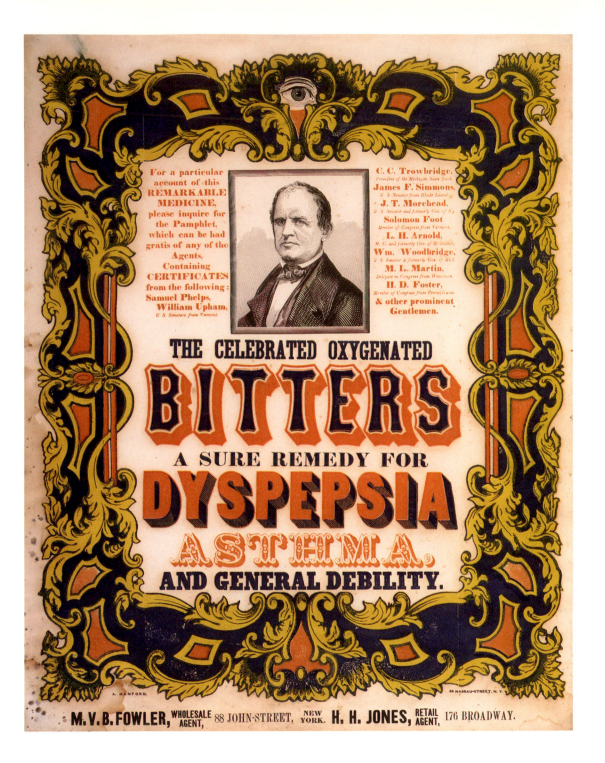

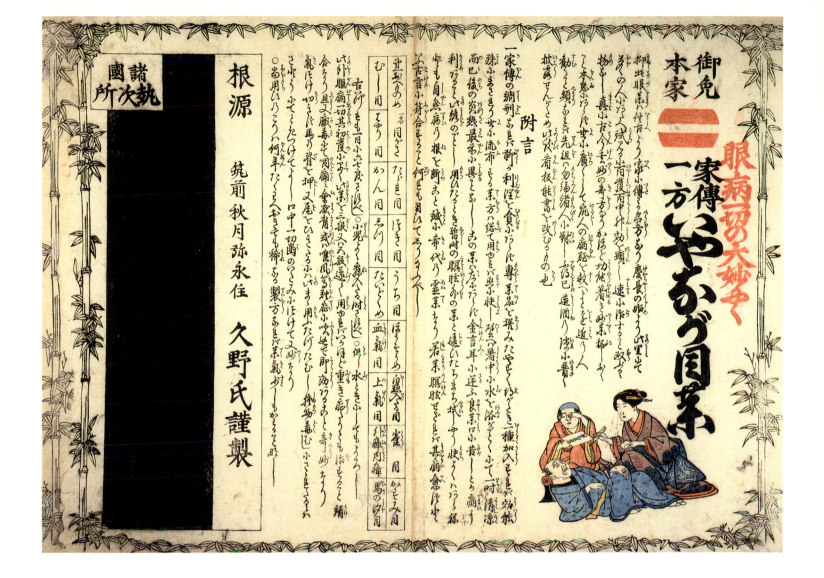

3
Homoeopathic Mutual Life
Insurance Company
Anonymous, American
c. 1880
Lithograph
26½ x 20″ (67.3 x 50.8 cm)
1981-114-29

The medical practice of homeopathy, introduced by the German
physician Samuel Hahnemann at
the close of the eighteenth century,
has two basic tenets. The first holds
that "like cures like" (*similia simili-
bus curantur*), or that diseases or
their symptoms are cured by agents
producing similar pathologic effects
in healthy individuals. The second
is that drug potency is enhanced
by infinitesimal doses, often meas-
ured in terms of millionths of full
strength. Nineteenth-century insurance firms were not convinced of the
validity of this approach to healing,
however, and demanded higher
premiums for patients not under
the care of orthodox, or allopathic,
physicians. Homeopaths resented
the actuarial implication that their
system of medicine was unduly
hazardous, and thus specialized
insurance firms, such as the
Homoeopathic Mutual Life Insurance Company, were established to
meet their patients' needs.

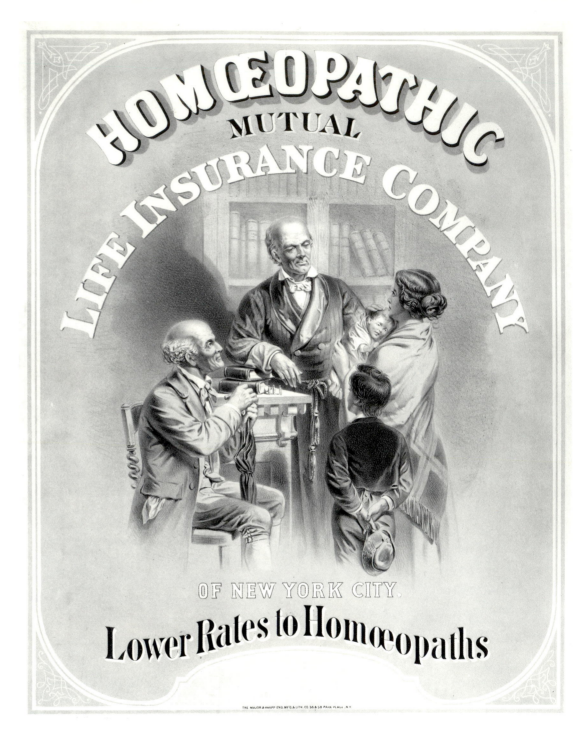

4
No-To-Bac
Maxfield Parrish (American, 1870–1966)
1890–1900
Color relief print
42 1/16 x 29 1/8″ (106.8 x 74 cm)
1981-114-36

The knight of No-To-Bac has slain his archenemy, Nicotine, in a poster that is as timely today as it was when it appeared almost one hundred years ago. No-To-Bac contained licorice, gentian, guaiac, and a salt, possibly ammonium chloride, and was prepared as a gum to be chewed. The pleasant demulcent action provided a substitute for smoking, but it was not successful with everyone. The knight was an image associated in all promotion for the product; he generally had short hair and a muscular torso labeled "King No-To-Bac." Here Parrish has varied the symbol to make him into a Roman warrior with long, flowing hair, but the inscriptions on the antagonists' shields remain the same.

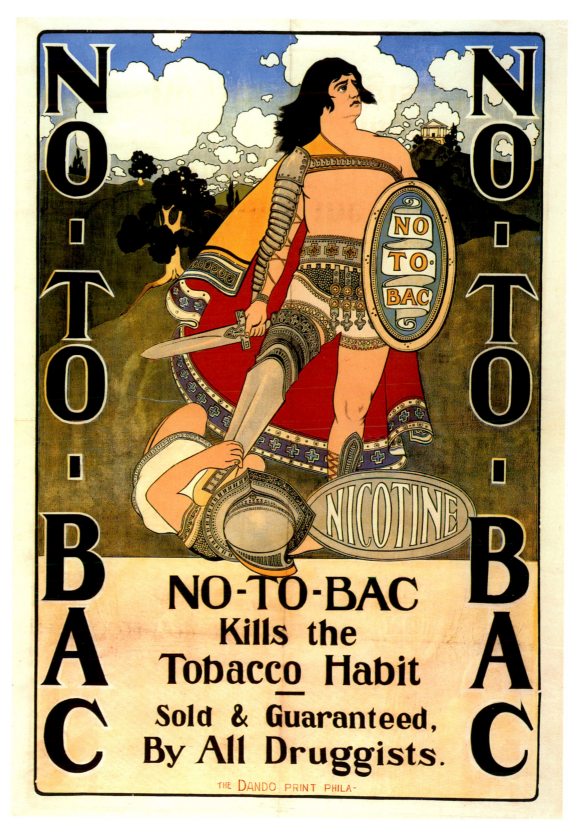

5
Fête Parisienne
Anonymous, French
1890 or 1902
Lithograph
23³⁄₈ x 15¹⁄₈″ (59.4 x 38.4 cm)
1981-114-24

Although cholera had been confined to Asia before 1830, improved communications and expanded travel by merchants, soldiers, and tourists led to several devastating pandemics in Europe and the Americas during the nineteenth and early twentieth centuries. This poster advertises the forthcoming Fête Parisienne to benefit cholera victims and their survivors. Its use of a somber gray illustration with a Pietà-like composition of woman and child, an anguished supplicating figure in the shadows, and a welcoming angel, is designed to elicit public sympathy and support. The poster is one of the first on a public health theme, for earlier nineteenth-century examples were almost exclusively advertisements for proprietary medicines.

6
Le Solitaire
Armand Jean-Baptiste Segaud
(French, born 1875)
1890–1900
Color lithograph
48¹¹⁄₁₆ x 34⁵⁄₈″ (123.6 x 88 cm)
Lent by William H. Helfand

A woman is about to annihilate a magnified microbe with an electrified rod known as Le Solitaire, an apparatus invented by L. de Boyères that was purported to cure all blood and nerve disorders. Charlatans such as De Boyères have always thrived on advances in technology, using electricity, radium, and even moon dust as the bases for their outlandish claims. Le Solitaire was not the first product of its sort, for it had been preceded by the metallic tractors patented by Elisha Perkins in 1796, which enjoyed great popularity in England until being exposed as fraudulent (see no. 36).

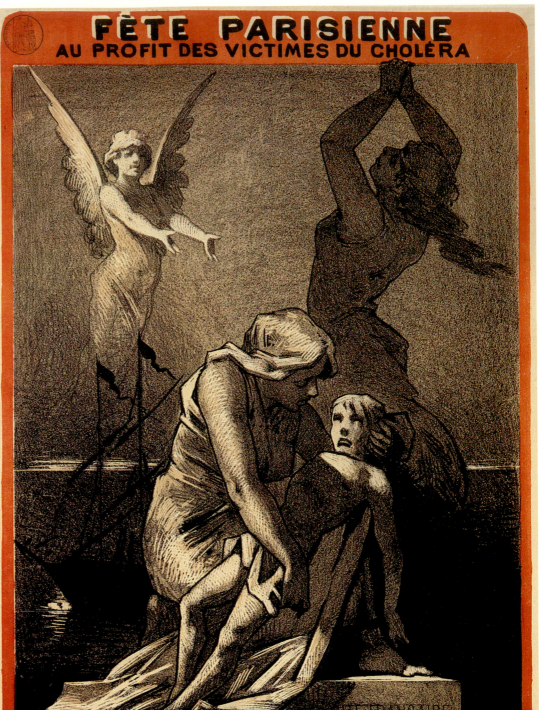

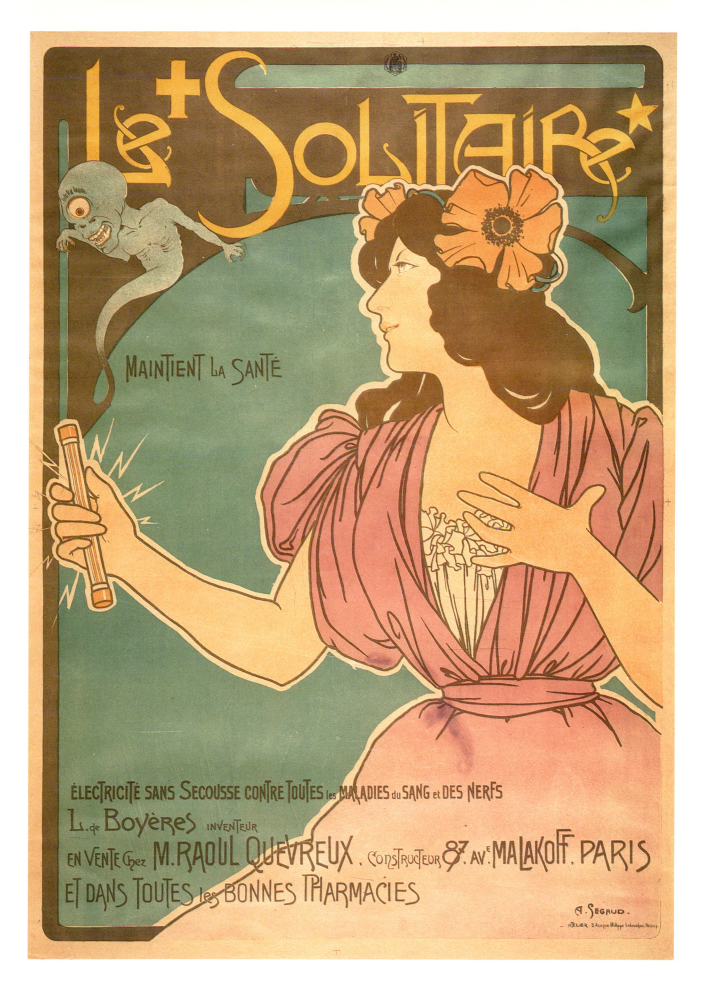

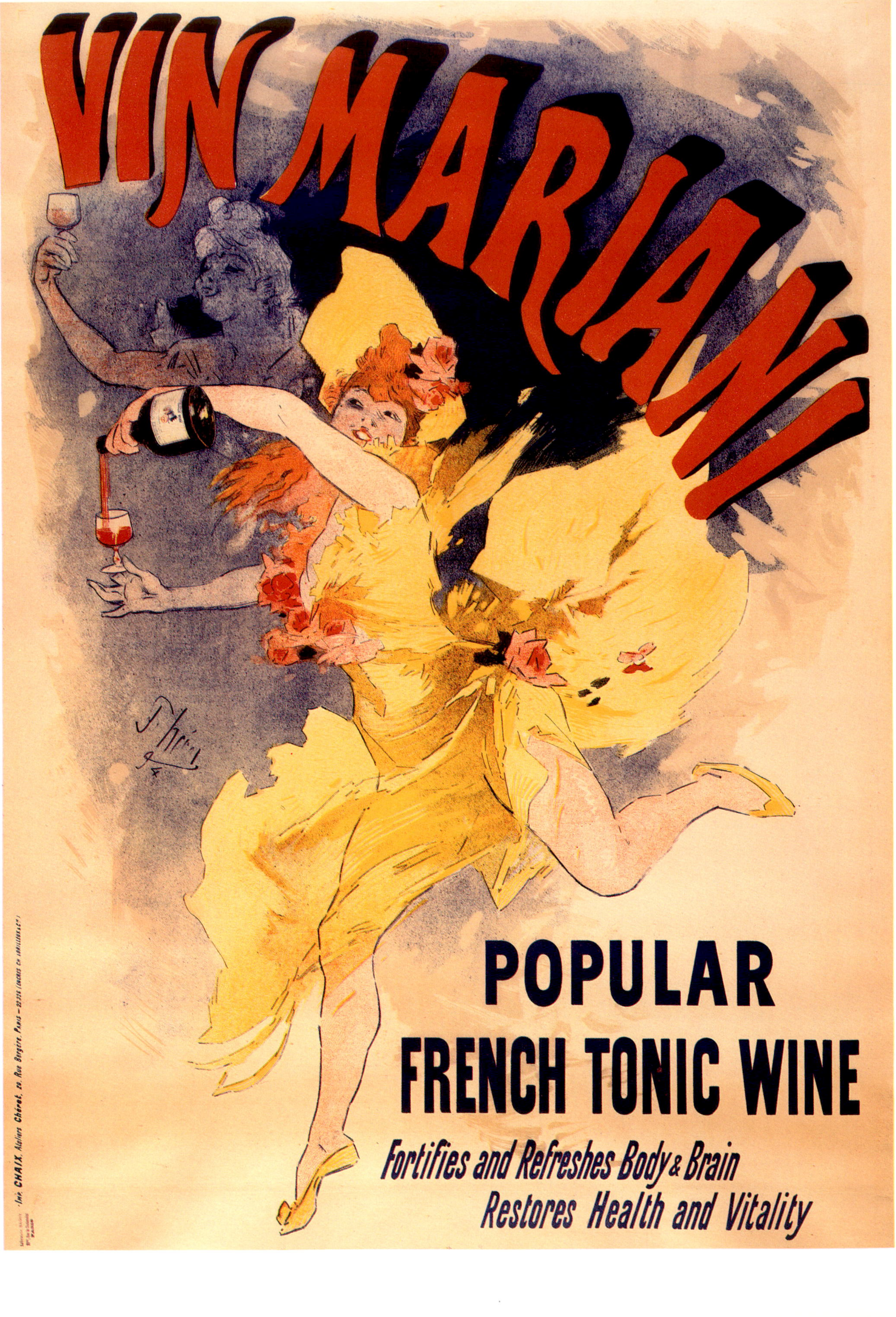
VIN MARIANI
POPULAR
FRENCH TONIC WINE
Fortifies and Refreshes Body & Brain
Restores Health and Vitality

7
Vin Mariani
Jules Chéret (French, 1836–1932)
1894
Color lithograph
49 x 34⅛" (124.5 x 86.7 cm)
Lent by William H. Helfand

Angelo Mariani developed the formula for his refreshing tonic wine shortly after the Franco-Prussian War of 1870–71, and, thanks to his marketing skills, it became one of the most widely recognized brands in Europe and North America in the years preceding World War I. Cocaine was the active ingredient of the product, which was prepared by steeping fresh leaves of the Peruvian bush *Erythroxylon coca* in "specially chosen" Bordeaux wine, in quantities of about two ounces of leaves per pint of wine. Chéret's poster shows two women, one pouring and the other in the background ready to drink a glass of Vin Mariani.

8
Pastilles Géraudel
Jules Chéret (French, 1836–1932)
1896
Color lithograph
22¾ x 15¼" (57.8 x 38.8 cm)
1989-69-5

The model navigating the dense snowfall illustrates one of several posters Chéret created for Pastilles Géraudel; each has the same ethereal woman (the model having been Madame Chéret) and the same slogan, "If you cough, take Géraudel's Pastilles." This phrase appeared in the English, French, and Italian versions of the poster, for the Géraudel firm was a major international advertiser at the turn of the century. The pastilles came in a small cylindrical container, an example of which is in the model's hand.

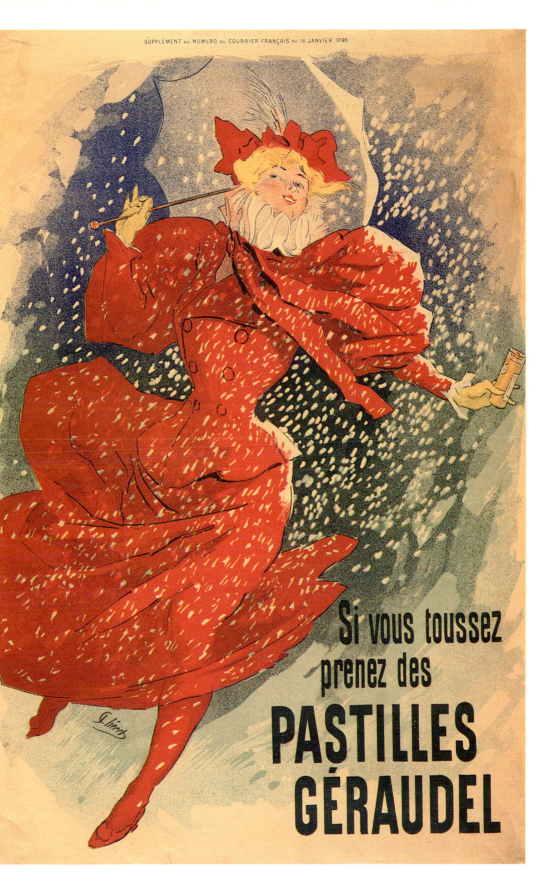

9

Amor vincit omnia (Love Conquers All)
Adolphe-Louis-Charles Crespin
(Belgian, born 1859)
c. 1895
Color lithograph
22³/₈ x 17¹/₁₆″ (56.8 x 43.3 cm)
1991-24-5

Crespin developed this image for Robert B. Goldschmidt, a professor of chemistry in Brussels who, among his many other accomplishments, had developed a pharmaceutical product known as Actiphos. Standing among varied chemical and pharmaceutical apparatus is a large black cat, in all probability an allusion to Goldschmidt's known affection for the animal. The bottles at the lower right, labeled for sulfur (S) and potassium hydroxide (KOH), represent a play on the French phrase *souffre et potasse*, in argot meaning "to study."

10

Ayer's Sarsaparilla
Anonymous, American
c. 1895
Color lithograph
40⁵/₁₆ x 29³/₈″ (102.4 x 74.6 cm)
1988-102-9

Dr. James Cook Ayer introduced his Sarsaparilla in 1848. While its principal advertised ingredient was the root of *Smilax officinalis*, the American sarsaparilla, this probably had no therapeutic value whatsoever; other vegetable drugs, such as queen's-root, yellow dock, and mayapple, produced the tonic effect for which the product was best known. Neither its plentiful quantity of glycerin, more than 50 percent of the volume, nor potassium iodide, an expectorant normally used to treat bronchitis and asthma, is known to produce the promised benefit "for the blood." The Ayer company advertised its products as widely as any nineteenth-century patent medicine firm, but this Sarsaparilla poster is unusual in showing an elderly man as a contented user.

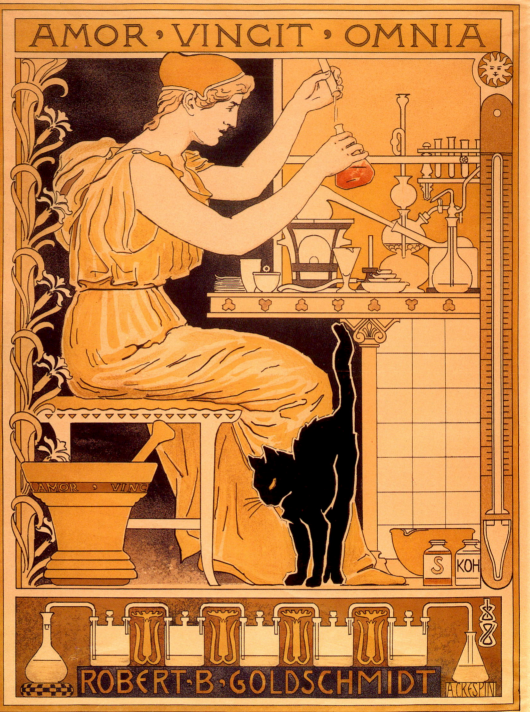

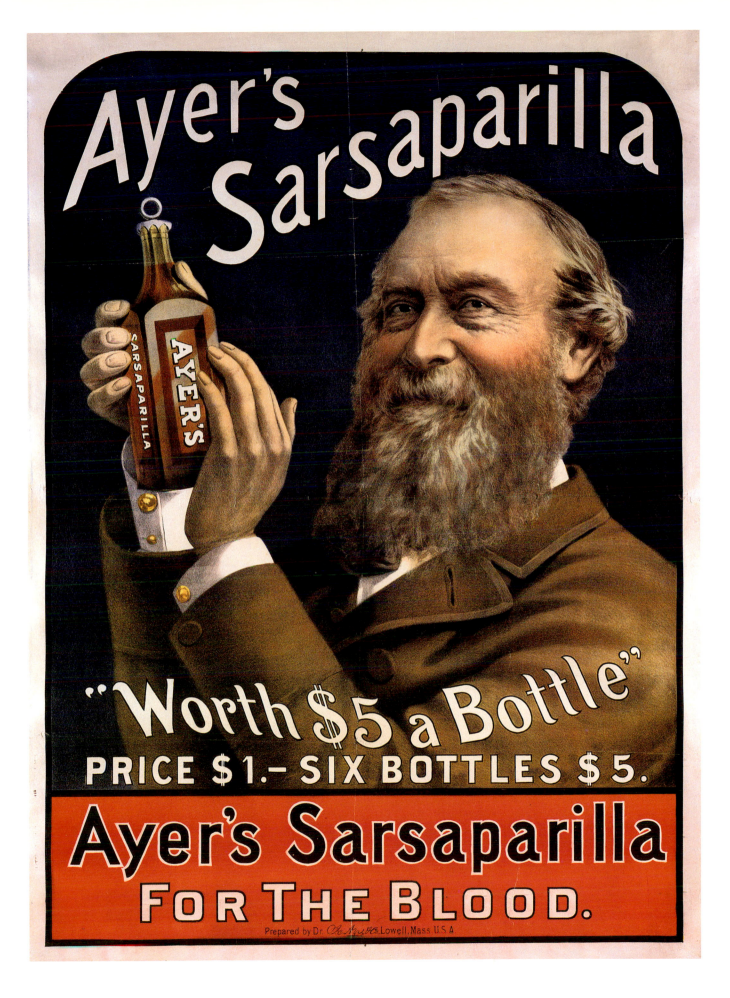

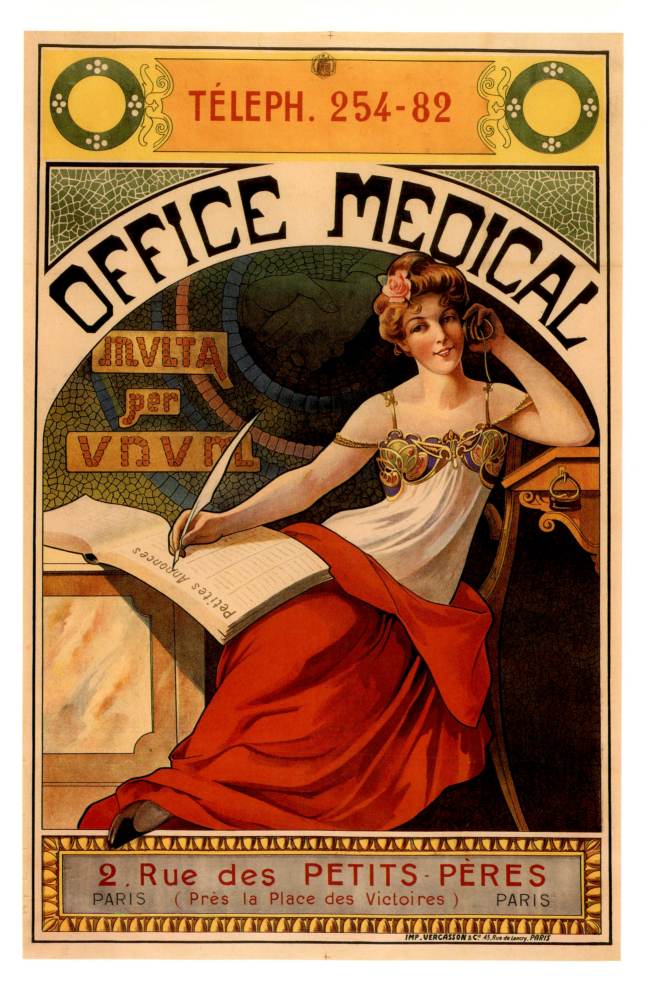

11
Office Médical
Anonymous, French
c. 1895
Color lithograph
45⅝ x 30¼" (115.9 x 76.8 cm)
Lent by William H. Helfand

The Office Médical in Paris was a service for placing classified advertisements for physicians in newspapers and magazines, and the Latin inscription, *multa per unum* (one for many), on this poster summarizes the purpose of the agency. An elegant receptionist is shown taking an order by telephone as she curiously—and anachronistically—writes with a quill pen. Placing advertisements by telephone was a novel concept in the late nineteenth century, and this poster accordingly gives particular importance to the service's telephone number. Such an image would surely have attracted a good deal of attention at the time.

12
Sífilis (Syphilis)
Ramón Casas (Spanish, 1866–1932)
1895
Collotype and color relief print
29¹¹⁄₁₆ x 13⁷⁄₁₆" (75.4 x 34.1 cm)
1979-137-1

It is no simple matter for artists to depict the causes of infectious disease; over time they have resorted to the use of imps, elves, gigantic crustaceans, snakes, enlarged microbes, and, in recent years, extraterrestrials. In this poster for a sanatorium for syphilis patients in Barcelona, Casas uses a snake crawling on the woman's shawl as a metaphor for venereal infection. Although the first truly effective antisyphilitic, Paul Ehrlich's Salvarsan ("606"), was not formally announced until 1910, fifteen years after this poster was published, the advertised sanatorium still promised an "unconditional and radical cure."

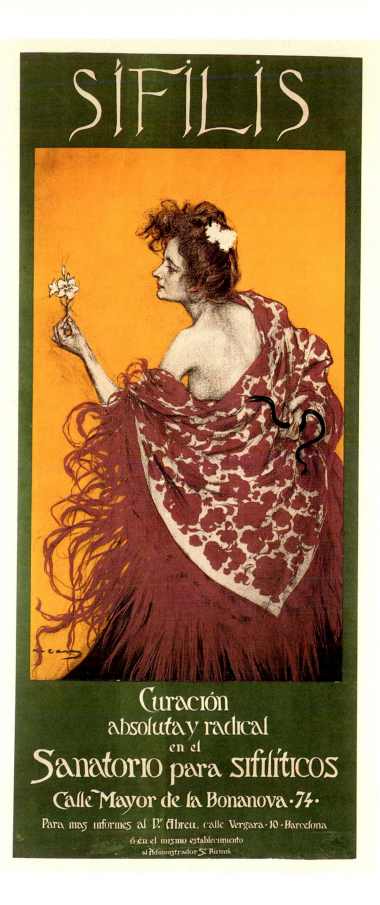

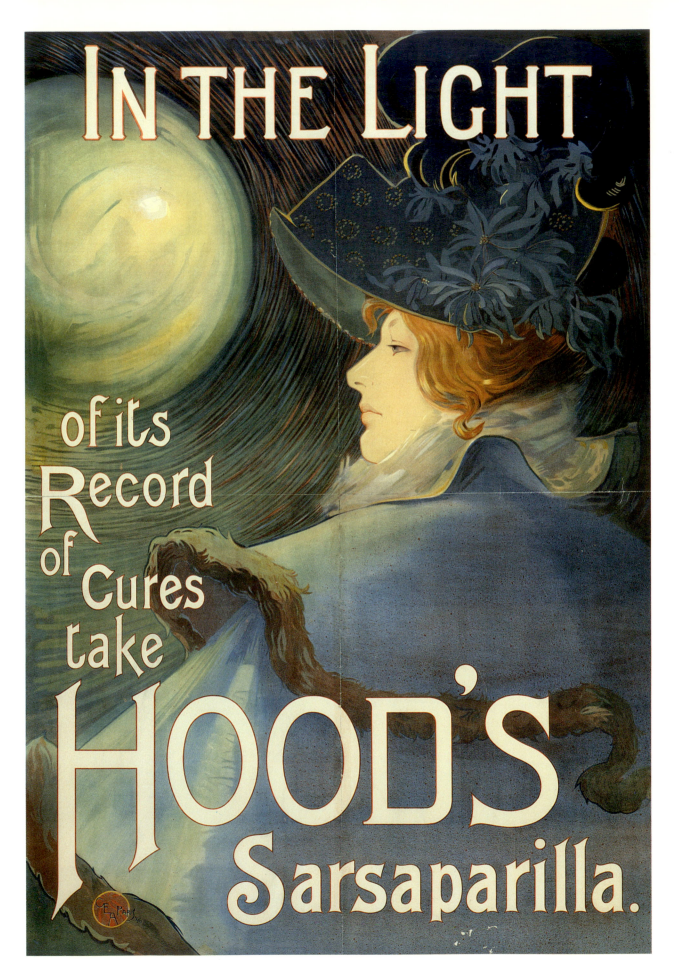

13

Hood's Sarsaparilla

C.E.A. (possibly French, n.d.)
1896
Color lithograph
42 x 29¼" (106.7 x 74.3 cm)
1977-47-1

Hood's Sarsaparilla was claimed to cure a variety of serious problems, including eczema, cancerous humors, catarrh, rheumatism, consumption, and dropsy. It contained about 18 percent alcohol and assorted herbs and roots such as sarsaparilla, licorice, and a drug resembling senna, which was largely responsible for its basic laxative effect. The poster does not focus on the product's indications, however, but urges its use "In the Light of its Record of Cures," a concept effectively reinforced by the model facing the light. Hood's Sarsaparilla had in fact been on the market for twenty years before this poster was published.

14

Esposizione d'igiene (Hygiene Exposition)

Adolf Hohenstein (German, active Italy, born 1854)
c. 1900
Color lithograph with pochoir
94⅛ x 46⅝" (239 x 118.4 cm)
1989-69-1

At the turn of the century Milan and Dresden, among other European cities, were hosts to annual hygiene exhibitions for which posters frequently were produced. Hohenstein's large poster, published for the 1900 exhibition in Naples, uses an image of an idealized family drinking from a pure mountain stream, identified as the *fons vitae* (the fountain of life), that offers the four requisites of good hygiene: light, air, water, and exercise.

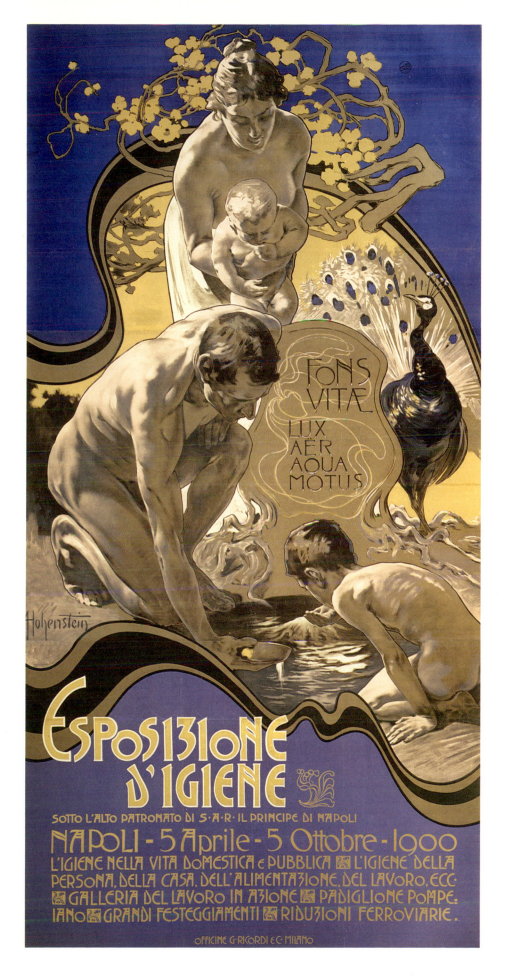

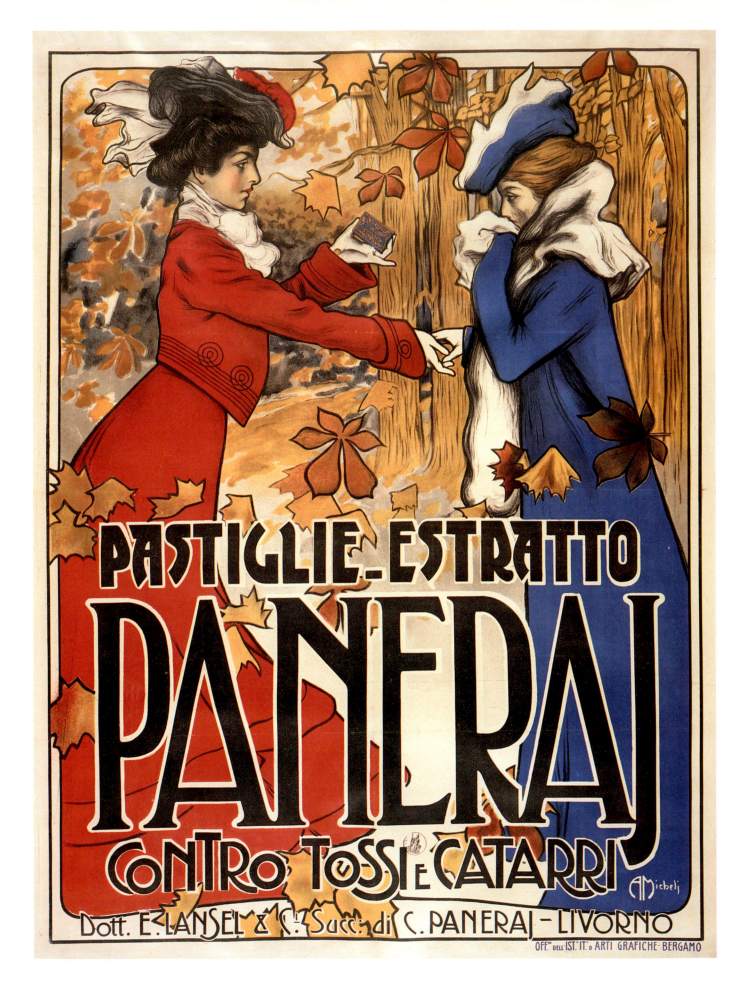

15
Pastiglie-Estratto Paneraj
Alberto Micheli (Italian,
1870–1905)
c. 1900
Color lithograph
50½ x 37¼" (128.2 x 94.6 cm)
1991-24-6

In this autumnal scene of two
women, one holds a handkerchief to
contend with a cold, while her friend
offers a package of Pastiglie-Estratto
Paneraj, which claims to be effective "against coughs and catarrhs."
The main ingredient in the pastilles
was concentrated lettuce juice,
but additional excipients probably
afforded topical relief as well.
Micheli's text is not integrated with
the illustration, but is superimposed
on its lower half almost as an after-
thought.

16
C. Degen & Cie
Fernand Schultz-Wettel (German,
born 1872)
1902
Color lithograph
24 x 17¾" (60.9 x 45.1 cm)
1988-102-124

The Degen company of Frankfurt
was a manufacturer of bandages and
dressings, examples of which can be
seen in the poster. Schultz-Wettel
has composed the scene in the style
of a *sacra conversazione* (holy
conversation) of Italian religious
painting, implying that the firm's
products possibly fulfilled more than
routine commercial purposes.

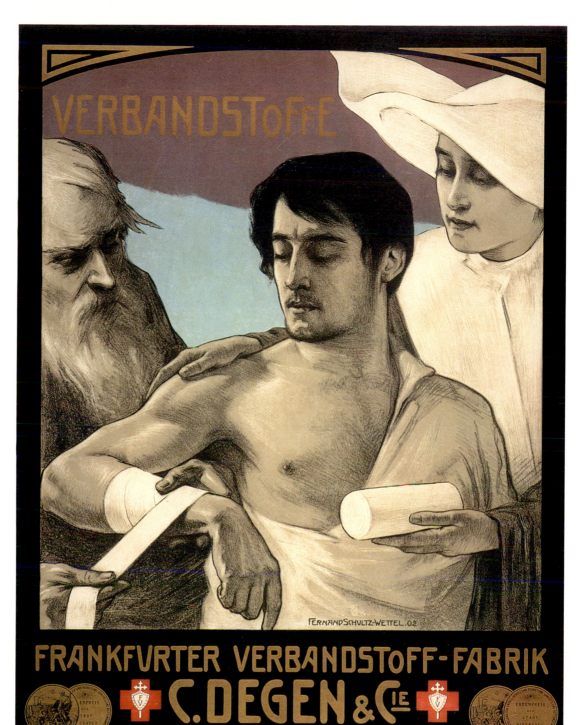

17
Katabexine
Leonetto Cappiello (French, born
Italy, 1875–1942)
1903
Color lithograph
55⅛ x 39 1/16″ (140 x 99.2 cm)
1988-102-54

The woman advertising Katabexine
appears to be in superb health, a
state obviously brought about by the
use of the product in her hand.
Katabexine, an effervescent tablet,
was recommended for all types of
cough as well as for bronchitis and
asthma. The elegant drawing, with
bright primary colors contrasted
against a black background, contains elements of Cappiello's style
that insured excellent visibility of
his posters, even from a long dis-
tance, making them especially
effective when mounted on exterior
walls.

18
Le Thermogène
Leonetto Cappiello (French, born
Italy, 1875–1942)
1909
Color lithograph
60½ x 45¼″ (153.7 x 114.9 cm)
1981-114-55

Le Thermogène has been on the
European market since about the
turn of the century. Never a popular
dosage form in the United States, it
is composed of soft cotton wadding
treated with capsicum, a blistering
agent that is responsible for the
product's activity when applied to
any part of the body where heat
would be beneficial. No advertisement in Le Thermogène's history has
had a greater impact than this
Cappiello poster with its fire-eating
circus performer holding the product close to his chest; it has become
an icon of creative advertising
imagery.

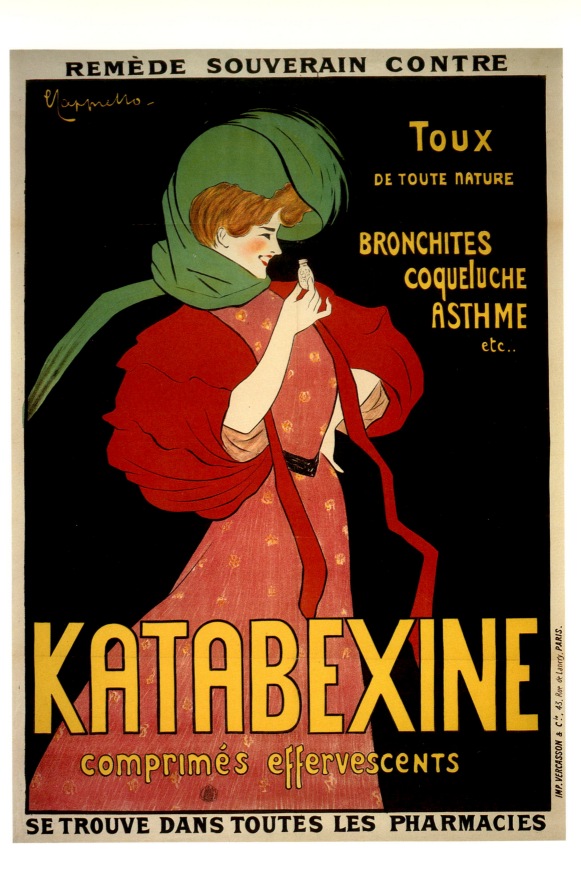

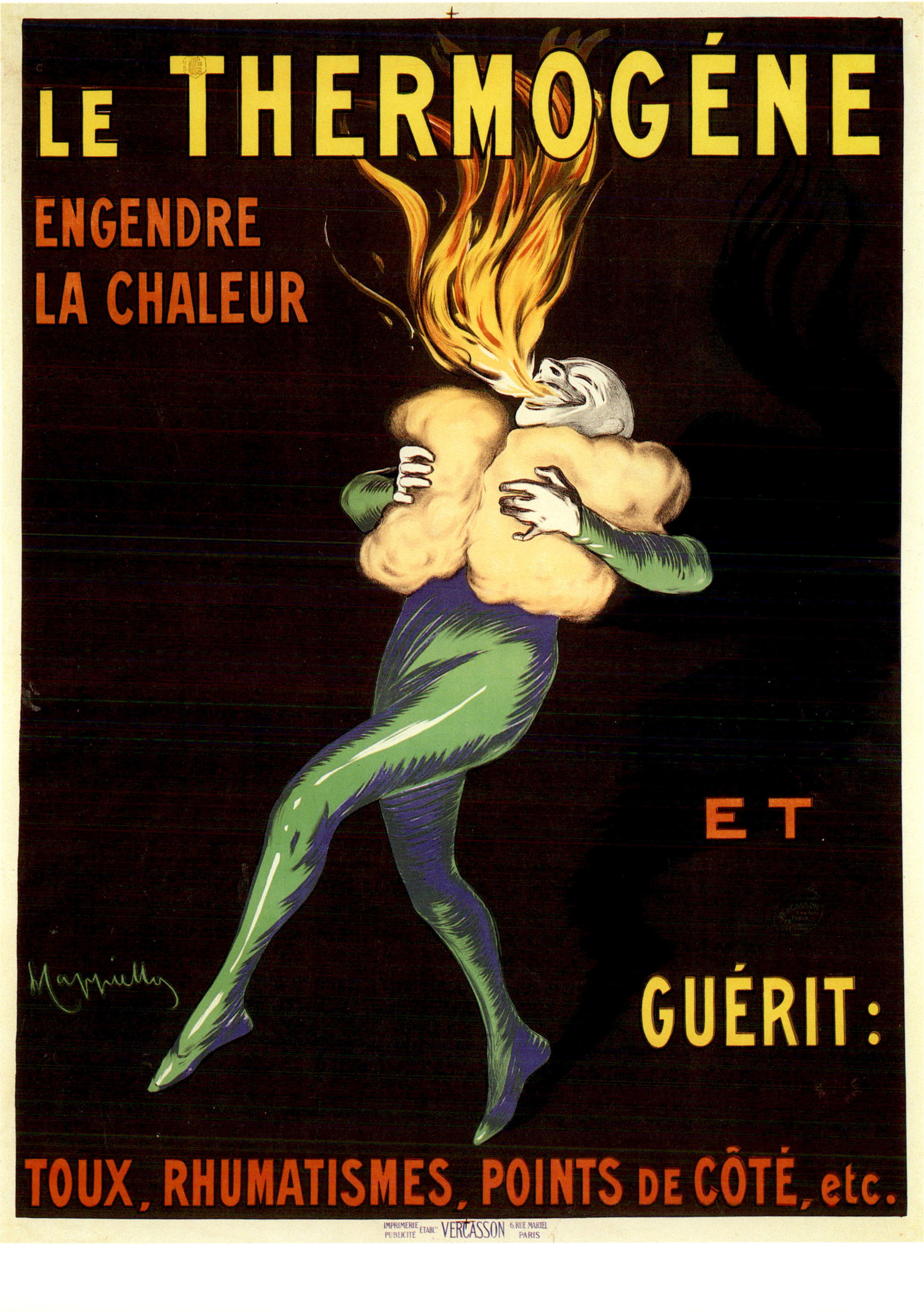
LE THERMOGÉNE
ENGENDRE
LA CHALEUR
ET
GUÉRIT:
TOUX, RHUMATISMES, POINTS DE CÔTÉ, etc.
IMPRIMERIE PUBLICITÉ ÉTABL[ts] VERCASSON 6, RUE MARTEL PARIS

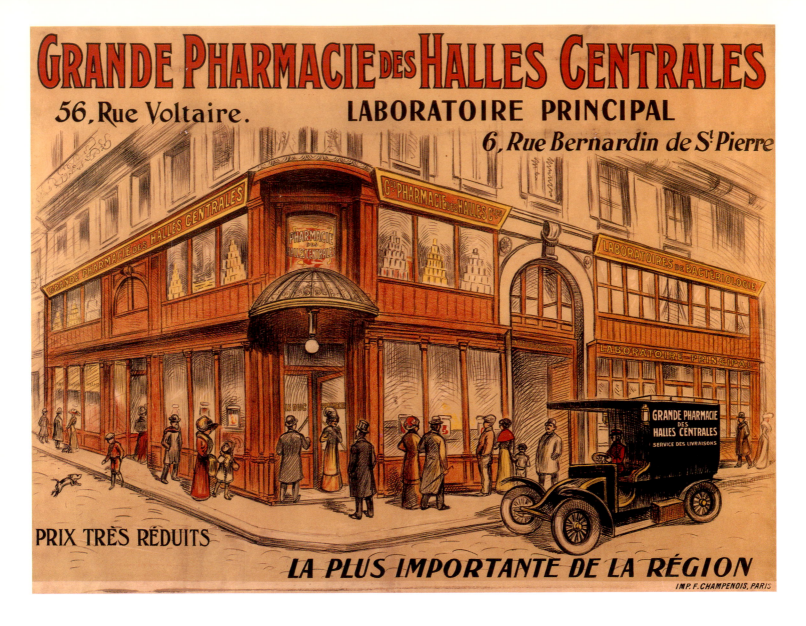

19

Grande Pharmacie des Halles Centrales
Anonymous, French
c. 1905
Color lithograph
46 x 62⅛″ (116.8 x 157.8 cm)
1977-47-2

Monsieur Le Duc was the owner of the Grande Pharmacie des Halles Centrales in Le Havre. His pharmacy fills the entire space of the poster; both the animated scene on the sidewalk and the delivery truck at the right attest to an active business. Until its destruction by Allied bombardment during the liberation of France in 1944, the facade remained as it is shown here; as recently as 1974 there was still a pharmacy, more modern in structure, on the site.

20

Dr. Dessauer's Touring Apotheke
Carl Kunst (German, 1884–1912)
c. 1910
Color lithograph
29⅞ x 19¾″ (75.9 x 50.2 cm)
1988-102-111

The poster advertises a first-aid kit, whose compact contents can be seen in the open box in the foreground. The kit seems to have had all the requisites for a country journey, including salves, antiseptics, and a plentiful supply of bandages, one of which is being used by the hiker.

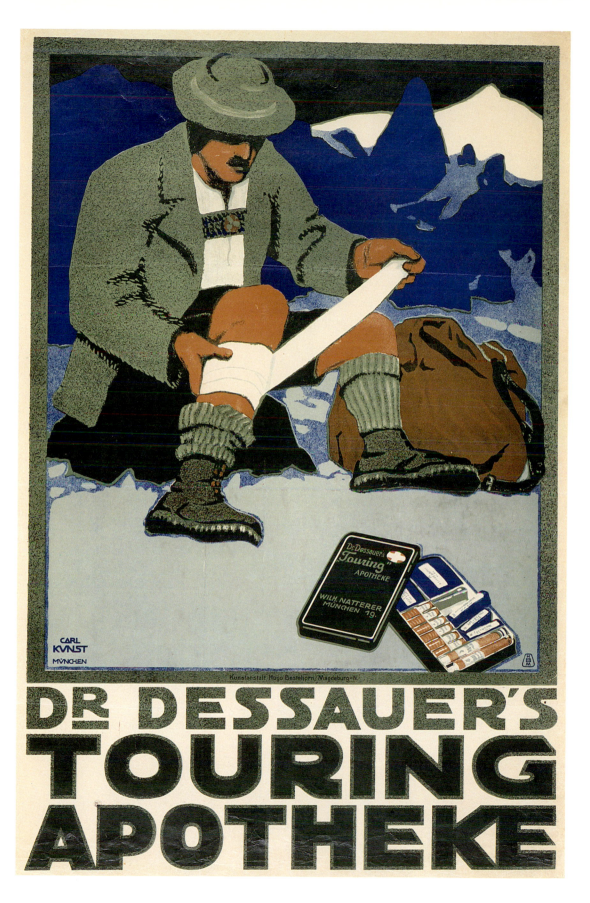

21
Sapho and **Détersif**
C. Morino Andreini (Italian, n.d.)
c. 1910
Color lithograph
93¹¹/₁₆ x 31⅝" (238 x 80.3 cm)
Lent by William H. Helfand

It is rare for a poster to advertise two products on a single sheet with no indication that the sections were to be separated. In this unusual example, the products do bear a slight relationship to one another, both being whiteners. The upper portion advertises Sapho, a dental powder, with a name possibly derived from that of the ancient Greek poet of Lesbos; the lower portion advertises Détersif, a powder to be added to the bath for whitening and softening the skin. Both illustrations are contained within an Art Nouveau decorative border, with appropriate typefaces well incorporated into the overall design.

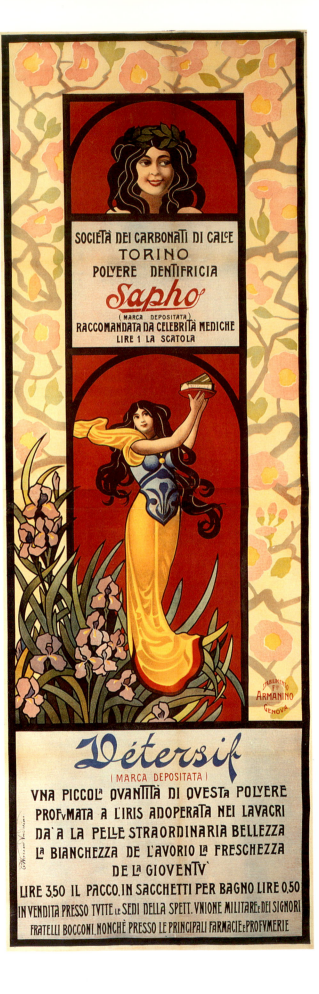

22

**Soldat, la patrie compte sur toi
(Soldier, the Country Relies on You)**
Théophile-Alexandre Steinlen
(French, 1859–1923)
1916
Lithograph
31½ x 23¹³/₁₆" (80 x 60.5 cm)
1988-102-127

Warnings against venereal disease are among the earliest subjects of twentieth-century public health posters. In this example Steinlen dramatically appeals to French soldiers to maintain their strength for their country and to resist those "seductions of the street" that carry with them the risk of exposure to an illness that is as "dangerous as war" and may lead to a "useless death without honor." The contrast between life, represented by a healthy soldier surrounded by laurel leaves and his country's flags, and death, symbolized by a skull and crossbones amidst withered branches and thorns, is reinforced by a gravestone-like tablet on which the impassioned warning is written. Reflecting the sensibility of the times, neither the word *syphilis* nor *gonorrhea* nor even *venereal disease* appears in the text.

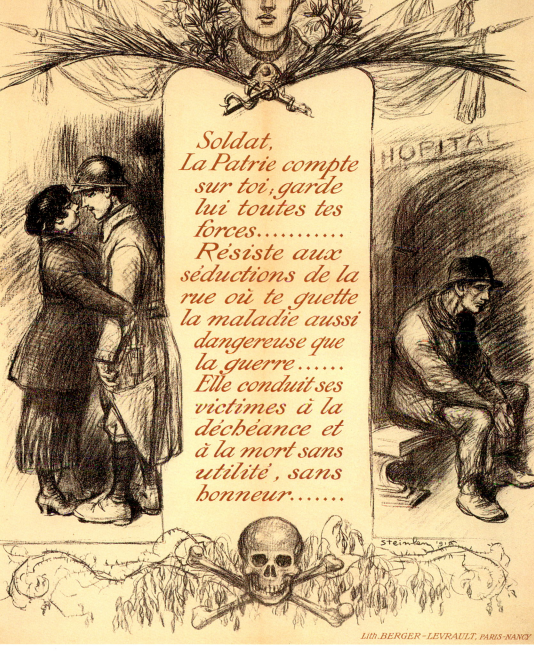

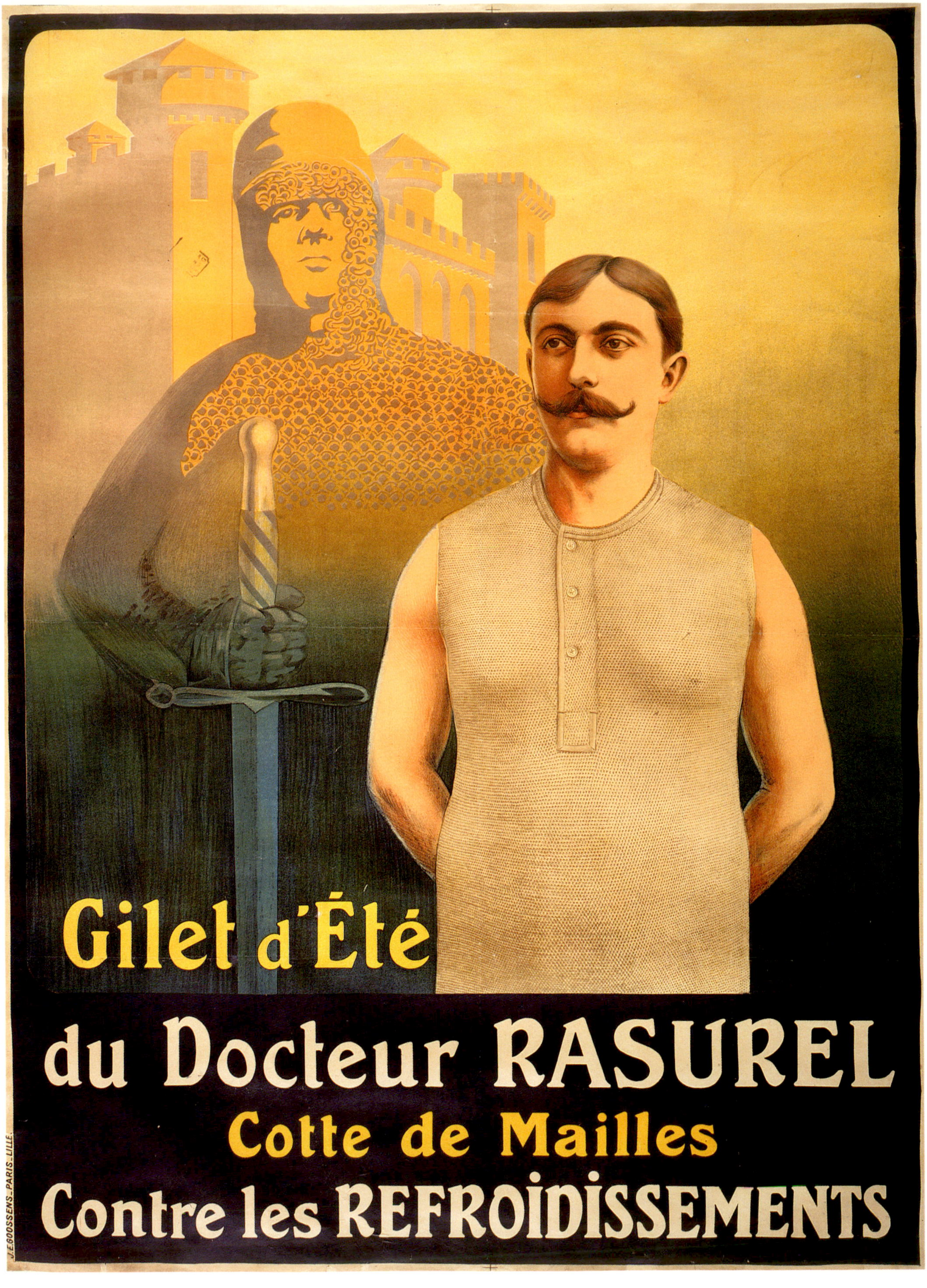
Gilet d'Été
du Docteur RASUREL
Cotte de Mailles
Contre les REFROIDISSEMENTS
J.E.GOOSSENS_PARIS_LILLE.

23
Gilet d'Eté du Docteur Rasurel
Anonymous, French
c. 1920
Color lithograph
62$^{13}/_{16}$ x 45$^{11}/_{16}$"
(159.5 x 116 cm)
1991-24-3

The moustached model wears a summer vest, one of many types of hygienic underwear manufactured by the Docteur Rasurel firm, a company still doing business in Europe. Promoted as a "coat of mail" similar to that worn by the knight in the background, it is in fact an early example of thermal fabric that one is advised to wear against sudden summer chills.

24
Un Grand Fléau: La Tuberculose
(A Great Scourge: Tuberculosis)
F. Galais (French, n.d.)
c. 1920
Color lithograph
62$^{11}/_{16}$ x 47$^{1}/_{2}$"
(159.2 x 120.6 cm)
1988-102-79

Practices that encourage rather than control the development of "a great scourge: tuberculosis" are shown in this crowded image that depicts the urban poor throwing refuse from windows, taking food from trash heaps, and drinking. Hovering over the scene is the shadowy, skeletal Angel of Death holding a scythe. Galais's poster was one of several commissioned by the Rockefeller Foundation to aid the overwhelming number of tuberculosis victims in France at the conclusion of World War I.

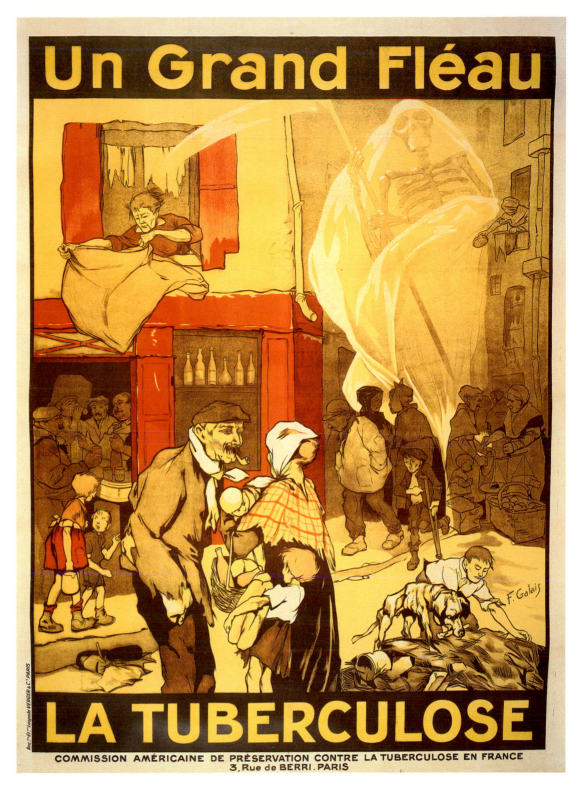

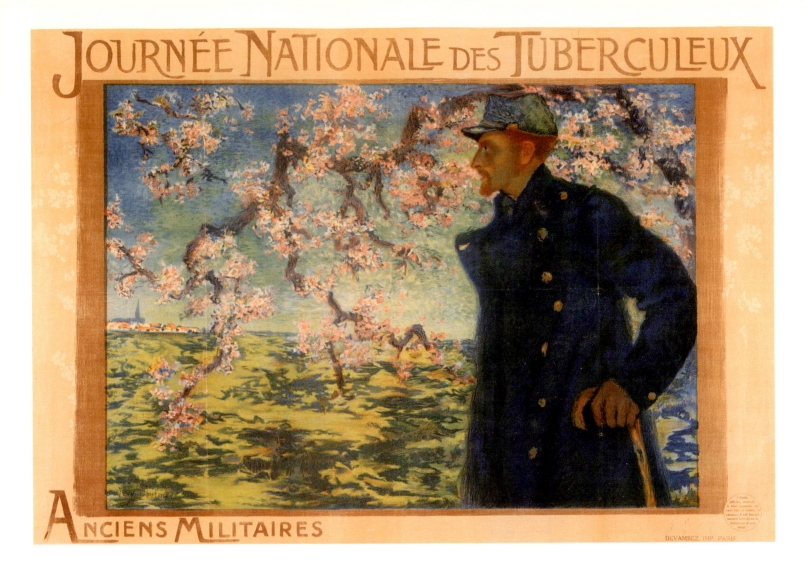

25

Journée nationale des tuberculeux (National Day for the Benefit of Tubercular Soldiers)
Lucien Lévy-Dhurmer (French, 1865–1953)
c. 1920
Color lithograph
32⅞ x 44¹⁵⁄₁₆" (83.5 x 114.1 cm)
1981-114-31

Lévy-Dhurmer's poster was produced for the Journée nationale des tuberculeux, an annual fundraising event for French servicemen afflicted with tuberculosis. It presents a sharp contrast between the lively, colorful flowers on the tree branches and the dark figure of the melancholy, emaciated soldier, supported by his walking stick. A note at the bottom of the poster admonishes the public to treat it with care and to understand that it is not for sale.

26

Italiani, aiutate la Croce Rossa nell'assistenza ai tubercolosi (Italians, Help the Red Cross to Cure Those with Tuberculosis)
Basilio Cascella (Italian, 1860–1950)
c. 1920
Color lithograph
39⅛ x 26⅞" (99.4 x 68.3 cm)
1988-102-56

The Red Cross nurse uses a small dagger to attack a globe-encircling monster, metaphorically representing tuberculosis. In contrast to this black, menacing evil, the nurse is dressed in white, which heightens the drama of the battle. The text pleads with Italians to "help the Red Cross to cure those with tuberculosis," such fundraising efforts having been a major activity of Red Cross agencies throughout the world in the years before World War II.

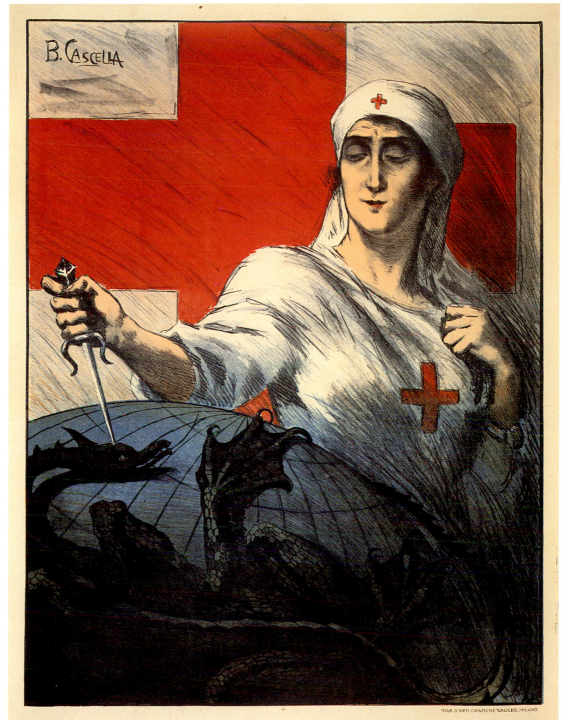

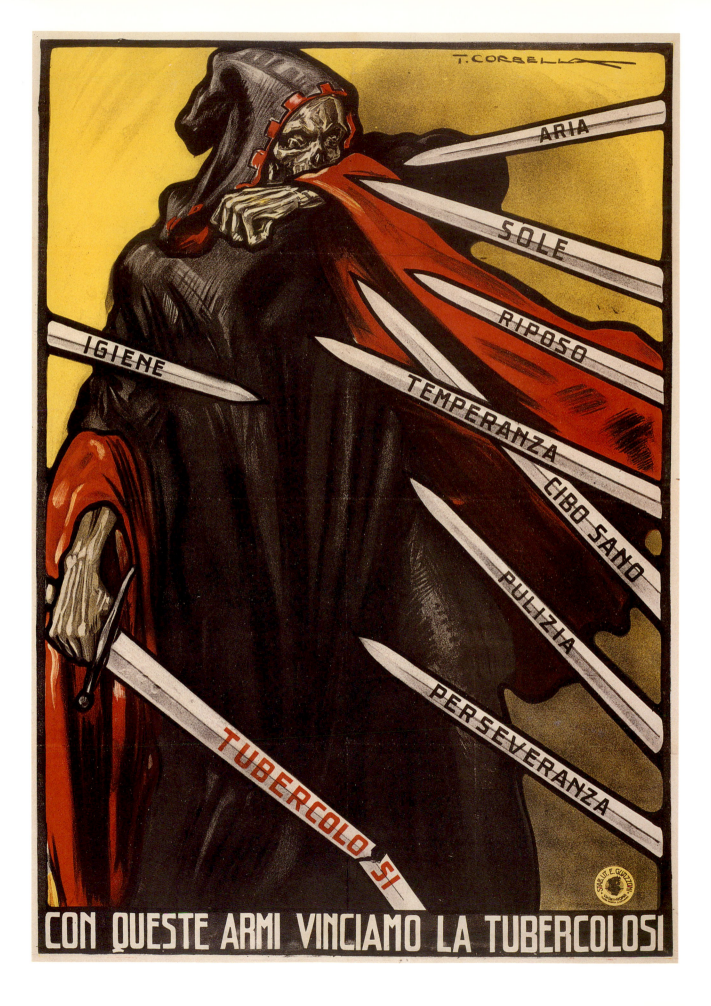

27
**Con queste armi vinciamo la
tuberculosi (With These Weapons
We Shall Conquer Tuberculosis)**
T. Corbella (Italian, n.d.)
c. 1920
Color lithograph
38¼ x 27" (97.2 x 68.5 cm)
1988-102-58

Swords bearing the means to attack
tuberculosis cause the foreboding
figure of the disease to cower. Corbella's skeletal image of the illness
holds a sword that has been broken
by the onslaught of the disease-
fighting weapons — good hygiene,
fresh air, sunshine, rest, temperance, proper food, cleanliness, and
perseverance. Together these forces
provide assurance that "we shall
conquer tuberculosis."

28
L'Embrocation Chanteclair
Michel Liébeaux (French,
1881–1923)
c. 1920
Color lithograph
24⅛ x 15¾" (61.3 x 40 cm)
1988-102-114

An embrocation is meant to be
rubbed on painful skin areas for
relief, but in his illustration the artist
implies that Chanteclair will do
much more. His muscular genie has
escaped from the bottle charged
with electricity, for the product is, as
the poster declares, "the developer
of athletes." The product claims also
that it "softens, fortifies, and electri-
fies," the last action in keeping with
the now-discarded belief that electricity had health-giving properties.

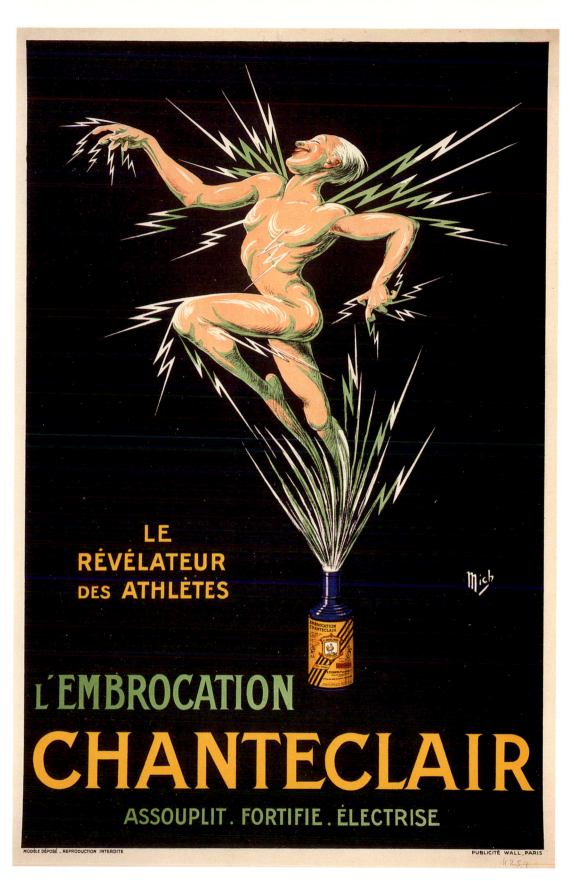

29
Pastilles Valda
Anonymous, French
c. 1930
Color lithograph
47³/₁₆ x 31⁵/₈" (119.8 x 80.3 cm)
1988-102-32

Although extensively magnified in the box held by the top-hatted salesman, Pastilles Valda are in reality small green lozenges with a pleasant, aromatic flavor. As with similar products, they have an antiseptic, decongestant, and demulcent action that promises to "take care of colds, coughs, and sore throats." The product is still marketed throughout the world, the design of its label having changed little since this lithograph was made.

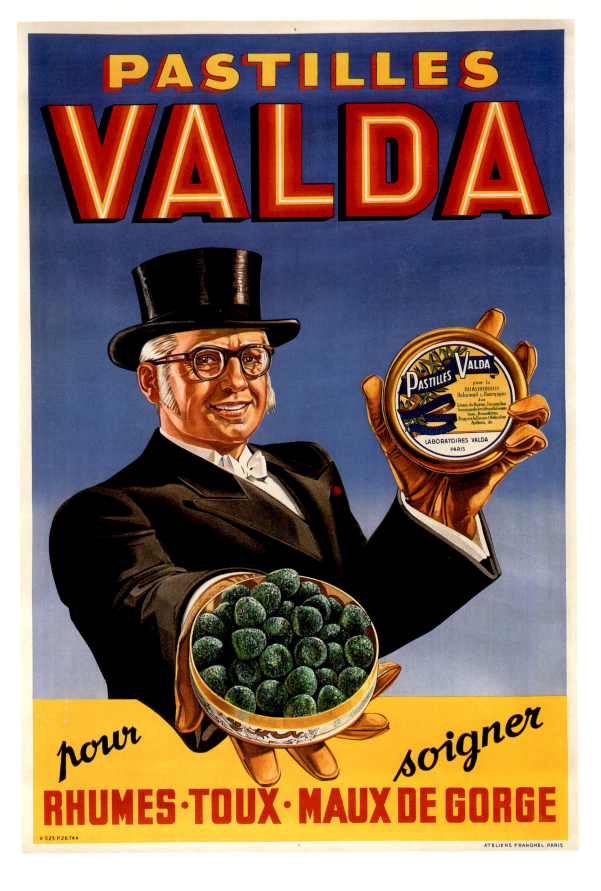

30
Marihuana: Weed with Roots in Hell
Anonymous, American
c. 1936
Color relief print
41³/₄ x 27⁵/₁₆" (106 x 69.4 cm)
1989-69-6

Although marihuana had long been in widespread use in the United States, it was not thought to be a serious health problem until the 1930s. But the Depression exacerbated fear of the effects of marihuana in certain areas of the country, particularly the South and West, and it began to be perceived as being as dangerous as heroin. The film *Marihuana: Weed with Roots in Hell* played upon this fear, vividly describing the depths of degradation the drug might produce. To entice the viewer to see this "daring drug exposé," this poster combines lurid descriptions of the "shame, horror, despair, . . . misery, weird orgies, . . . [and] unleashed passions" that marihuana can cause with vivid illustrations of the users themselves. Accuracy was not a major consideration, however, for marihuana is shown being injected in addition to being smoked as a cigarette or in a pipe.

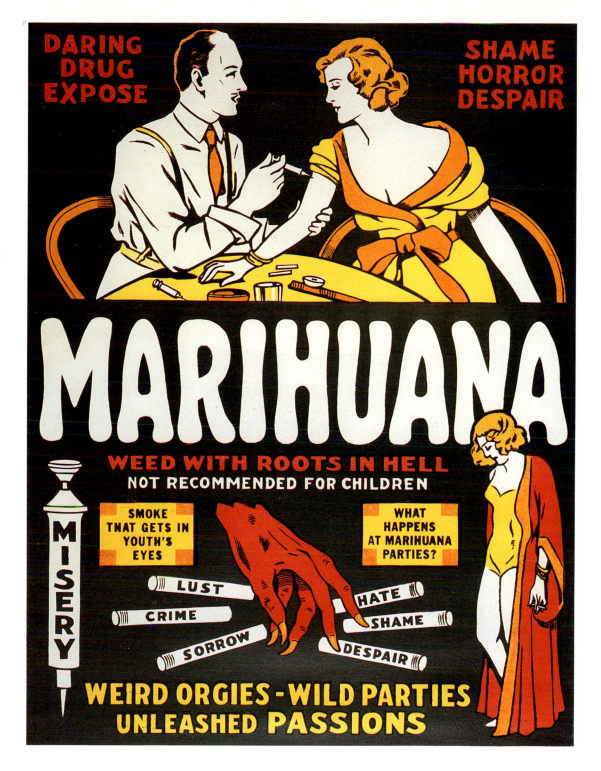

31

AIDS Prevention
David Lance Goines (American,
born 1945)
1985
Offset lithograph
24 x 17" (60.9 x 43.1 cm)
1989-69-3

The contemporary San Francisco
artist David Lance Goines created
this poster, which was sold to raise
funds for the AIDS prevention program at the University of California's
Student Health Service. His image
of a snake curled around an apple,
however, aroused some controversy
among those who felt that it implied
an association between the disease
and the concept of sin. Transmission
of the AIDS virus in the United
States is predominantly by sexual
practices, but can also occur
through the infected needles of
intravenous drug users and the
transfusion of contaminated blood.

32

**A Gala Night for Singing: A Benefit
for AIDS**
Paul Davis (American, born 1938)
1985
Color halftone
30¼ x 21½" (76.9 x 54.6 cm)
1989-69-4

The first posters dealing with the
worldwide AIDS epidemic began to
appear in the early 1980s; hundreds
have since been published on varied
aspects of the disease, including
treatment and prevention, that
continue to defy solution (see no.
31). Although in this example the
illustration does not pertain to the
illness itself, Davis's poster, like
those used in earlier campaigns to
combat cholera (see no. 5), tuberculosis (see nos. 25, 26), and polio,
was designed to help raise funds to
benefit disease victims.

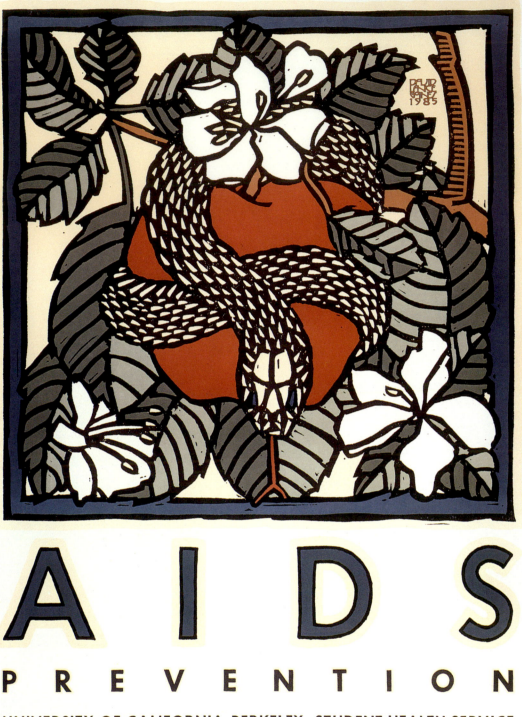

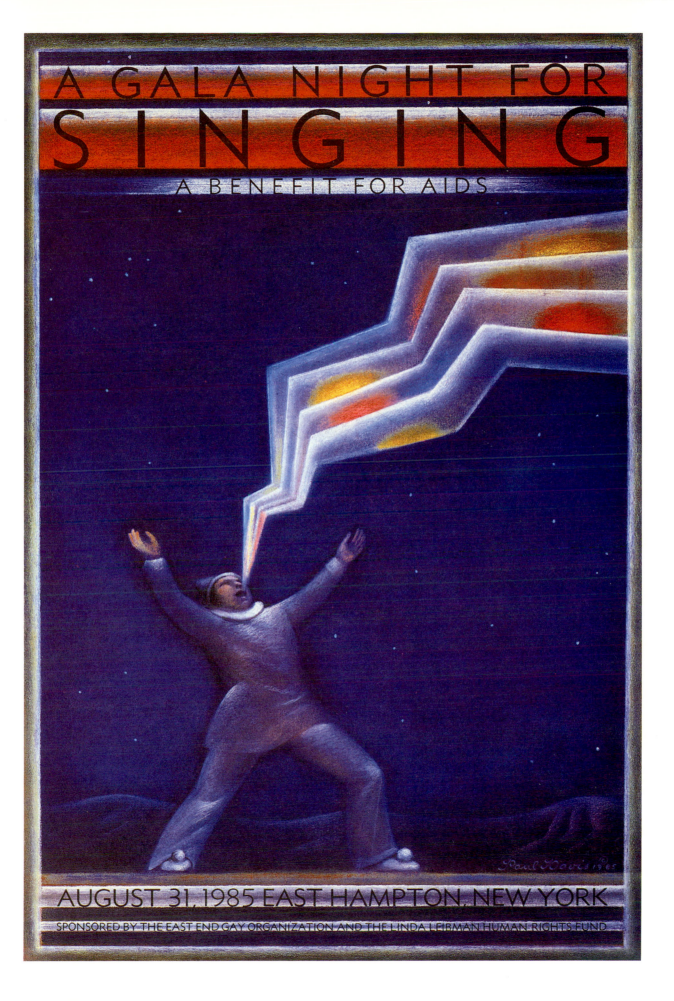

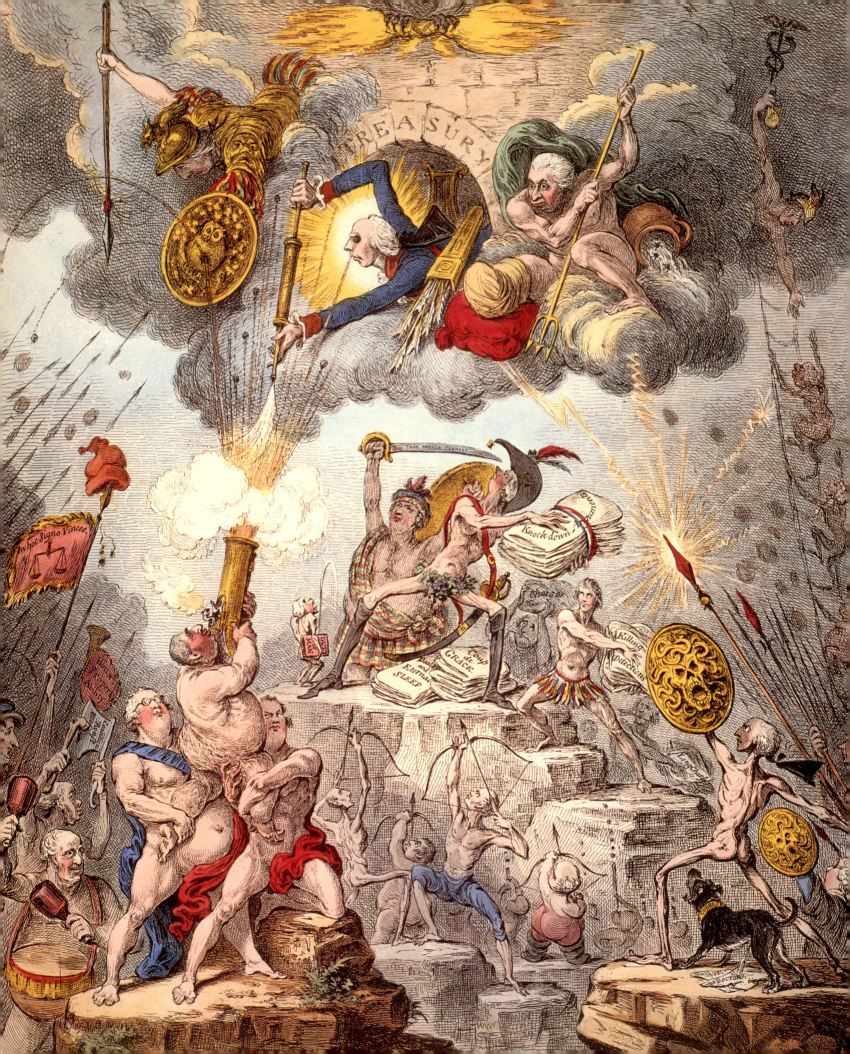

The Caricature of Medicine   Judith Wechsler

Detail of *Confederated-Coalition; or The Giants Storming Heaven* by James Gillray (no. 39)

Caricature is the art of exaggerating or distorting features and events for satirical purposes, either social or political. The term was derived from the word *caricare* (to load, charge, or exaggerate), which was coined in late-sixteenth-century Italy and describes portraits that are not only exaggerated but also designed to attack. Caricature marks a radical departure from the norms of beauty and decorum; it is the antithesis of the classical ideal. But before the artistic laws, theories, and values could be broken, they first had to be established.[1] During the Italian Renaissance Western standards of beauty and pictorial composition were systematically defined, and caricature, as we know it, developed then as a kind of counterdiscourse. Italian charged portraits first appeared in England in the 1730s, and were known as *caricatures*.[2]

Caricature also relates to the tradition of the grotesque in art, as exemplified in ancient masks, medieval gargoyles, and the marginalia of manuscripts. Distorted and phantasmagoric figures have long fascinated artists, and can be seen in the works of Leonardo da Vinci, Lucas Cranach, Pieter Brueghel the Elder, Hieronymus Bosch, Jacques Callot, Francisco Goya, and James Ensor, among others. The subject of illness or deviation from health necessarily entails the rendering of the abnormal and the grotesque. It is one of the few subjects that invites deformation and makes the departure from classical or ideal beauty a necessary condition.

Genre scenes, with their frank renderings of life, were also significant for the development of caricature. The paintings and prints of sixteenth- and seventeenth-century Holland, Flanders, and Germany were closer to everyday experience than those of the classical tradition. So too were the political prints made during the Hundred Years' War (1337–1453), when moralizing broadsides and picture pamphlets were dispersed to a wide public. These popular images with their political and social messages intersected with the charged Italian portraits to form the basis of English and French caricature.

1. For a discussion of the psychology of caricature and its links with aggression, see Ernst Kris and E. H. Gombrich, "The Principles of Caricature"; reprinted in Ernst Kris, *Psychoanalytic Explorations in Art* (New York, 1952), pp. 189–203. For history and theory, see Werner Hofmann, *Caricature from Leonardo to Picasso* (New York, 1957).

2. *The Oxford English Dictionary* cites the use of the word *caricatura* as early as 1682 and 1690. In *English Political Caricature to 1792: A Study of Opinion and Propaganda* ([Oxford, 1959], p. 12), M. Dorothy George quotes the use of the term by the duchess of Marlborough in 1710. See also Victoria and Albert Museum, London, *English Caricature, 1670 to the Present: Caricaturists and Satirists, Their Art, Their Purpose and Influence* (London, 1984), pp. 13–14.

Michel Melot asserts that caricature could only come to the fore with the support of a bourgeois culture, "the class that supplied the audience and the infrastructure for caricature";[3] an active commerce in prints; and a taste for genre images, democratized portraits, and engravings of current events. All of these conditions existed in both mid-eighteenth-century England and revolutionary France.

Caricatures appeared in eighteenth-century England initially as prints, issued in series or singly, and were limited to a rather educated and affluent audience. These prints could be purchased from printsellers and publishers, and were also lent out for an evening's entertainment. In France and England, mass circulation of caricatures, essentially to the middle class, did not occur until the nineteenth and early twentieth centuries with their publication in such satirical journals and albums as *La Caricature, Le Charivari, Le Journal amusant, L'Eclipse, La Lune, L'Assiette au beurre, Punch,* and *Vanity Fair* (see nos. 54–57, 62–66, 68, 69).

Medicine, perhaps more than any other profession, has been used for a variety of purposes in caricature. Pharmacies and other medical settings have appeared for more than 250 years in the political caricatures of England, France, and the United States, as William H. Helfand has noted.[4] Graphic satire using medical metaphors for sick and healthy societies emerged in the eighteenth century, when public health became a social priority and medicine as a profession assumed a new importance. Doctors had increasing presence and power in academic societies and in the political realm,[5] and medical consultation served as a parallel to political debate.[6] Despite the advances in the medical profession, however, the range of available treatments remained quite limited through the mid-nineteenth century, and thus not surprisingly ironic comparisons associated "the reputation of politicians with the charlatan figure of the medical practitioner."[7] Scenes of quackery prevailed, perhaps due to the overlap among the healing functions of barbers, surgeons, doctors, alchemists, sorcerers, astrologers, and apothecaries, professions not clearly defined before the mid-eighteenth century; even in the nineteenth century the distinctions among them were sometimes nebulous.[8]

The themes of medical caricature include allegories, usually as a commentary on politics; illness and disease; practice-malpractice; doctors and apothecaries; and pharmaceutics and cures, both metaphoric and practical. Relatively few caricatures focus on medical issues or practices as such; more frequently, medical themes and subjects are used as social and political allegories. For example, bleeding may be used to comment on financial problems, cathartics may symbolize the need to rid the political system of its impurities,[9] and the human body may stand for the body politic. Michel Foucault has observed that "the 'body'—the body of individuals and the body of populations—appears as the bearer of new variables."[10] The beleaguered nation is often pictured as an ailing patient, its legislators as doctors, and political solutions or practices as false cures. The use of these and

3. Michel Melot, "Caricature and the Revolution: The Situation in France in 1789," in Grunwald Center for the Graphic Arts, Wight Art Gallery, University of California, Los Angeles, *French Caricature and the French Revolution, 1789–1799* (Los Angeles, 1988), p. 73.

4. William H. Helfand, "The Pharmacist in British Political Prints," *Pharmacy in History,* vol. 31, no. 2 (1989), p. 52.

5. Michel Foucault, "The Politics of Health in the Eighteenth Century," in Michel Foucault, *Power/Knowledge: Selected Interviews and Other Writings, 1972–1977,* ed. Colin Gordon (New York, 1980), pp. 176–77.

6. Kate Arnold-Forster and Nigel Tallis, *The Bruising Apothecary: Images of Pharmacy and Medicine in Caricature* (London, 1989), pp. 8–9, 52.

7. Ibid., p. 52.

8. Janet S. Byrne, "Prints of Medical Interest," *The Metropolitan Museum of Art Bulletin,* vol. 5, no. 8 (April 1947), pp. 211–12.

9. William H. Helfand, *Medicine & Pharmacy in American Political Prints (1765–1870)* (Madison, 1978), pp. 14, 23.

10. Foucault, "The Politics of Health," p. 172.

other medical symbols provides the viewers with immediate connection to their own experiences.

Medical caricatures employ a number of devices to convey their message, including the use of recognizable motifs and compositions in altered and unexpected circumstances to produce new meanings. André Gill's *The Delivery* (no. 63) is an example of such a quotation; in a parody of Eugène Devéria's painting *The Birth of Henry IV* (Musée du Louvre, Paris),[11] it shows Louis Adolphe Thiers, the president of the republic, delivering France's baby. James Gillray's *Confederated-Coalition; or The Giants Storming Heaven* (no. 39) is a play on Baroque compositions. Ronald Paulson has observed that "every Gillray caricature is a comment upon the French *and* English norm of art."[12]

Caricature often works on a principle of juxtaposition or opposition: beauty is countered by deformity, or in medical caricature, health and wholeness are contrasted with disease and decrepitude. This is seen in Thomas Rowlandson's etching *Dropsy Courting Consumption* (no. 41), which shows an obese man on his knees before an emaciated woman. A further contrast is suggested by the placement of this improbable couple in a setting of classical architecture and sculpture.

There is an interesting relationship between the metaphoric language of pain and its representation in caricature. Jonathan Miller's application of the term "the pantomime of complaint" to the way in which patients indicate pain with their hands is useful to consider when studying caricatures.[13] In satirical prints pain is commonly personified as demons that attack the body. George Cruikshank, in *The Cholic* (no. 46), exteriorizes pain by picturing devils pulling each end of a rope wrapped around the waist of an agonized woman. In his *Blue Devils* (no. 47), which has been interpreted as a scene about depression, a man is beleaguered by demons representing his tormenters. This device still appears in advertisements for palliatives such as headache remedies and ointments for sore muscles.

Despite the advances in medicine in the major cities, bloodletting, purging, and clystering were widely prescribed for almost any sickness through the mid-nineteenth century.[14] These treatments are commonly applied allegorically in caricatures, as in Cruikshank's *Radical Quacks Giving a New Constitution to John Bull* (no. 45). Emblems also had metaphoric value. The clyster, or enema syringe, was a shorthand means of illustrating the administration of something either positive, such as advice, or harmful, such as oppressive taxation. A related theme depicts "some person or group prescribing or administering some remedy for the ills or problems of the nation."[15]

The clyster, which appears as an emblem for material purges in political prints from the United States and England but most extensively in those from France, had "obscene and phallic overtones" as well.[16] Albert Boime notes that "the anal origins of the term *charger*, to caricature, symbolizing the heaping of satiric dirt on the subject-victim, should be clear."[17] Scatological references in political caricature are the subject of several other studies.[18] Freud's

11. Isabelle Compin et al., *Catalogue sommaire illustré des peintures du Musée du Louvre et du Musée d'Orsay*, vol. 3, *Ecole française, A–K* (Paris, 1986), repro. p. 223.

12. Ronald Paulson, *Representations of Revolution (1789–1820)* (New Haven, 1983), p. 211.

13. Jonathan Miller, *The Body in Question* (New York, 1978), p. 33.

14. Theodore Zeldin, *France, 1848–1945*, vol. 1, *Ambition, Love and Politics* (Oxford, 1973), pp. 23–24.

15. William H. Helfand, "Medicine and Pharmacy in French Political Prints," *Transactions and Studies of the College of Physicians of Philadelphia*, 4th ser., vol. 42, no. 1 (July 1974), p. 21. Other medical and pharmaceutical emblems also had metaphysical value. The mortar and pestle represented governments, proposals, or political initiatives being broken or destroyed. See Helfand, "British Political Prints," p. 52.

16. Helfand, "French Political Prints," p. 17.

17. Albert Boime, "Jacques-Louis David, Scatological Discourse in the French Revolution, and the Art of Caricature," in Grunwald Center, *French Caricature*, p. 73.

18. See Ernst Kris, "The Psychology of Caricature" (1935); reprinted in Kris, *Psychoanalytic Explorations in Art*, pp. 173–88. See also James Cuno, "Introduction," in Grunwald Center, *French Caricature*, pp. 13–22.

concept of aggression, as set forth in his *Wit and Its Relation to the Unconscious* (1905), is often cited in this context:

Where a joke is not an aim in itself — that is, where it is not an innocent one — there are only two purposes that it may serve, and these two can themselves be subsumed under a single heading. It is either a *hostile* joke (serving the purpose of aggressiveness, satire, or defence) or an *obscene* joke (serving the purpose of exposure).[19]

Medical caricatures often have sexual overtones as well.[20] For example, Charles Maurin's *Aesculapius: Truffles for the Doctor and Drugs for the Patient* (no. 67) shows a well-heeled doctor proffered a steaming plate, while the reclining nude woman is offered medicine. Two covers from *L'Assiette au beurre* depict other aspects of the medical profession from an unfavorable perspective. In *The Pharmacists* by Démétrius Emmanuel Galanis (no. 69) an apothecary flirts with a woman, and in *The Doctors* by Jules-Abel Faivre (no. 68) a doctor nuzzles up to the back of an ugly older woman. The features of the doctor may well have anti-Semitic connotations in the wake of the Dreyfus affair.[21]

The moral force and bite of caricature, addressed to social and political issues, were developed in England beginning in the mid-eighteenth century. William Hogarth, who is considered the father of English caricature, advanced the interests of his profession by the copyright act he obtained in 1735.[22] He developed narrative etchings as a new satirical genre: his modern moral subjects that were made in the service of social reform. In his series "A Harlot's Progress" and "Marriage à-la-Mode," doctors are pictured as quacks.[23] Hogarth's influence is apparent in the moralizing social and political subjects and the focus on human behavior seen in the work of other English and French caricaturists.

The so-called golden or classic age of English caricature (early 1780s to the early part of the first decade of the 1800s) is perhaps best represented by the work of James Gillray, who is considered the first professional political cartoonist. It was he, for example, who invented the image of "Little Boney" for Napoleon, the first figure to be universally caricatured. Medical themes are represented in a number of his prints, such as *Doctor Sangrado Curing John Bull of Repletion* (no. 37), in which England is being bled to death. Other Gillray prints show dubious medical inventions and procedures, as in his *Metallic-Tractors* (no. 36) and *Comfort to the Corns* (no. 35). M. Dorothy George points out that after 1811, political prints were "relatively few and uninspired" (Gillray had become insane). Caricaturists focused on the Regency; events abroad were neglected.[24]

Caricature first flourished in France during the revolution, and medical themes were common.[25] The French caricatures were not quite as vicious and brutal in their depictions, however, as were their contemporary British equivalents. After the revolution, the widespread use of lithography; the increasing mechanization of the printing press, imported from England in the 1820s,

19. Sigmund Freud, *Jokes and Their Relation to the Unconscious,* ed. and trans. James Strachey (New York, 1960), pp. 96–97. The earlier English translations of this work were published as *Wit and Its Relation to the Unconscious.*

20. Isador H. Coriat, "The Psychology of Medical Satire," *Annals of Medical History,* vol. 3, no. 4 (Winter 1921), pp. 403–7.

21. On anti-Semitic caricature of the time, see Phillip Dennis Cate, "The Paris Cry: Graphic Artists and the Dreyfus Affair," in Norman L. Kleebatt, ed., *The Dreyfus Affair: Art, Truth, and Justice* (Berkeley, 1987), pp. 62–95.

22. Hogarth's Act, as it came to be known, secured engravers a copyright for their designs and thus protected their work from pirating by printsellers. See George, *English Political Caricature to 1792,* p. 111.

23. See Joseph Burke and Colin Caldwell, *Hogarth: The Complete Engravings* (London, 1968), pls. 138, 195.

24. M. Dorothy George, *English Political Caricature, 1793–1832: A Study of Opinion and Propaganda* (Oxford, 1959), pp. 128–29.

25. Helfand ("French Political Prints," p. 14) cites examples that appeared as early as 1565.

which doubled production while halving the cost; the founding of several journals devoted to the caricature; and the demographic growth of Paris led to the further popularity and dissemination of French caricature. People turned to prints and popular illustrated books for guidance in a rapidly changing urban environment. The interest in physiognomy and phrenology, the study of the physical signs of inner states, contributed to the vocabulary of caricature.[26] Focus on physical traits, central to the program of physiognomy, was an essential strategy of medical caricature.

Doctors and medicine continued to play a role in French political and social caricature into the nineteenth century, particularly during the monarchy of Louis-Philippe of 1830–48 (see nos. 54–57). In the French legislature of 1789, the first in which the bourgeoisie was represented, doctors served in large numbers. Theodore Zeldin points out that in 1848 there were some 1,550 doctors in Paris, 300 of whom were decorated with the Legion of Honor. The principal support of these physicians, who were "offering every variety of cure,"[27] came from the fees they charged the rich, and their financial and political success depended upon "nepotism, favoritism, camaraderie . . . carried to the highest degree."[28] Many doctors resorted to selling quack cures to augment their incomes, but genuine economic security was achieved by obtaining a part-time official appointment, which made them almost civil servants.[29] A contemporary text, *Les Français peints par eux-mêmes,* published in Paris in 1840–42, noted that when a doctor "has the misfortune to be nothing, either by one's titles or employments, one may still establish one's self as Homoeopathist, Phrenologist, Somnambulist, or Magnetiser."[30]

Because nineteenth-century French caricaturists were subjected to censorship laws of increasing stringency, they used doctors for veiled attacks on the government and as tropes for political manipulation and dishonesty. Physicians thus came to stand for a government that bled the nation and offered dubious cures.

Honoré Daumier, the leading French caricaturist of the nineteenth century, produced over four thousand lithographs, about one hundred of which had medical themes showing doctors, dentists, surgeons, nurses, oculists, hypnotists, homeopaths, phrenologists, pharmacists, and quacks.[31] His prints were published in such satirical periodicals as *La Caricature* (see nos. 54–57), *Le Charivari,* and *Le Journal amusant,* and had subscriptions and sales of about three thousand an issue. The readership was predominantly from the middle class, the very people who were the brunt of Daumier's satire.

One of Daumier's early political caricatures that used medical symbolism is *The Court of King Pétaud* (no. 55), in which a parade of supplicating ministers, one wielding a huge enema syringe, approach Louis-Philippe on his throne. Most of Daumier's prints with medical content are social rather than political, due to the censorship laws that prevailed for about thirty of the forty years that he was working.[32] Documenting the cholera epidemic, he shows its effect in one of his illustrations for the book *Némésis médicale* (no. 59), for

26. See Judith Wechsler, *A Human Comedy: Physiognomy and Caricature in 19th Century Paris* (Chicago, 1982).

27. Zeldin, *France*, vol. 1, p. 25. "The doctors, far from ignoring the quacks and the theorists, engaged in constant polemic with them, and the medical press attacked and ridiculed every idea, new and old, and every personality in the same slanderous and uninhibited way as the political papers" (ibid., p. 26).

28. Edouard Charton, *Guide pour la choix d'un état* (Paris, 1842), p. 387; quoted in ibid., p. 31.

29. Ibid., pp. 31–32.

30. Translated as L. Roux, "The Physician," in Jules Janin et al., *Pictures of the French: A Series of Literary and Graphic Delineations of French Character* (London, 1840), p. 77.

31. Helfand, "French Political Prints," p. 15.

32. Ibid., p. 16.

which he made thirty wood-engraved vignettes.[33] Daumier also did three oils and six drawings of scenes from Molière's *Le Malade imaginaire* (the play was first produced in 1673),[34] as well as several other drawings of doctors and patients.[35] There was a long French literary tradition of attacks on doctors, most notably in the writings of Molière, Montaigne, and Voltaire. These texts formed a background of opinion for Daumier and other French caricaturists who used medical subjects: they shared a low opinion of doctors and lawyers.

Caricatures, rooted as they are in a time, place, and culture, need to be decoded. Satirical images convey specific messages that for the most part contemporaries, familiar with the characters and events depicted, can read at a glance. When modern audiences examine eighteenth-century English or nineteenth-century French caricatures, however, the full range of associations is not accessible without explanatory notes and an understanding of the conventions of representation from which the satires deviate. Caricatures rely to varying degrees on texts to clarify their meaning. Frequently words are incorporated into the images in "balloons" that issue from the mouths of the characters, a device that dates back to late medieval illustrations and to paintings of the Annunciation, and continues in contemporary comic books.

Caricature, unlike most painting, works on a principle of opposition. Beauty is countered by deformity. In caricatures concerning medicine, it is the contrast of health and wholeness with disease, deformity, decrepitude. The doctor is depicted, for the most part, as a "healer" who harms, and is likely a quack. The body, individual or social, is not shown as an ideal or as a vehicle of pleasure, but rather as a field for struggle and contention, signaling distress.

Even when we lack precise information about the subjects, caricatures can still be viewed and read for social history, artistic skill, and amusement. The delectation that caricatures afford through both their inventive forms and their moral messages elevates the best of them from what Charles Baudelaire calls the level of the "significative comic," with its reference to the specific, to that of the "absolute comic," with all its fantasy and creativity.[36]

33. The text was written in rhyme by François Fabre, who was a doctor and pioneer in medical journalism, secretary of a medical society, and editor of *Clinique des hôpitaux* and *Gazette des hôpitaux.* A drawing of the subject also exists. See K. E. Maison, *Honoré Daumier: Catalogue Raisonné of the Paintings, Watercolours, and Drawings,* vol. 2, *The Watercolours and Drawings* (Greenwich, Conn., 1967), p. 244, no. 733 (pl. 288).

34. Maison, *Honoré Daumier,* vol. 1, *The Paintings* (Greenwich, Conn., 1968), pp. 133–34, nos. I-153, I-154 (pls. 130–31), pp. 173–74, no. I-223 (pl. 141); vol. 2, *The Watercolours,* p. 140, no. 405 (pl. 137), p. 151, no. 445 (pl. 152), pp. 160–61, nos. 475–76 (pls. 160–61), p. 162, no. 480 (pl. 162), p. 163, no. 485 (pl. 165).

35. Ibid., vol. 2, pp. 138–39, nos. 399–404 (pls. 134–37); p. 140, nos. 406–7 (pls. 137–38).

36. See Charles Baudelaire, "Of the Essence of Laughter, and Generally of the Comic in the Plastic Arts" (1855); reprinted in Charles Baudelaire, *Selected Writings on Art and Artists,* trans. P. E. Charvet (Harmondsworth, England, 1972), p. 161.

I am grateful to Carin Kloppers for her bibliographic research for this essay, and to Karen Kennedy for her careful checking of sources.

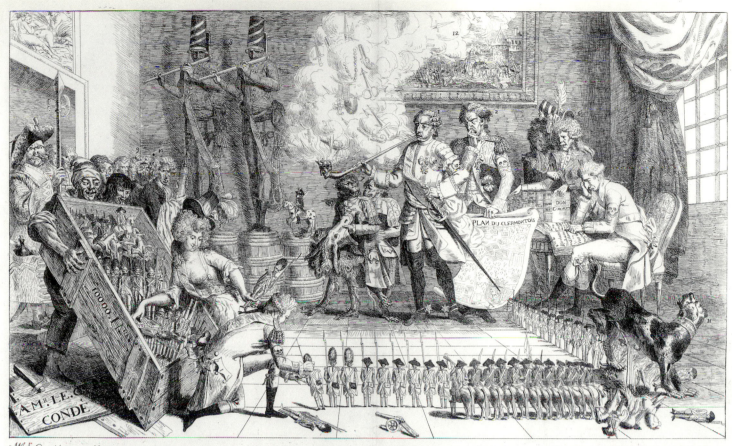

Grande Armée du cidev.r Prince de Condé

1 Mgr. Condé dans son Boudoir ou Château de Worms
passant en Revue l'armée formidable qui lui a été
envoyée de Strasbourg par la Diligence (*) On le voit
fumant sa pipe de laquelle s'exhalent en fumée
les Armes destinées à accomplir ses vastes Projets
2 Deutschamps son Écuyer méditant l'attaque
3 & 4 Mlle Condé jadis abb.e de Remiremont aide Major
déballant les Soldats & les passant au cidevant Duc
D'Enghien qui les dresse & les range en Bataille

5. Mr. Bourbon parcourant le Registre d'Enrôlement
6. Mme M.... ce Vivandiere de l'Armée
7. Les deux Pages de sa hautesse
8. Les heiducs sur des Barils demonitions jouant la fanfare
9 & 10. Un Médecin & un Appoticaire accourant à la
nouvelle hydrophobie du Grand Contre Révolutionnaire
11. Buttord en passant renverse un Escadron
12. Tableau représentant Worms réduit par les
françois en 1689

33

Grande armée du cidev[an]t Prince de Condé (The Grand Army of the Former Prince de Condé)
Anonymous, French
1791
Etching
16¹/₁₆ x 20½" (40.7 x 52 cm)
(plate)
16⁷/₈ x 21⁷/₈" (42.9 x 55.6 cm)
(sheet)
1988-102-25

Louis Joseph de Bourbon, prince de Condé, one of many émigrés who had left France to escape the Revolution, is shown in his château in Germany studying the resources that will enable him to restore the monarchy to his country. But he can only muster toy soldiers, and equally unreal guns and other armaments appear solely in the smoke from his pipe that covers a battle painting. A

physician and an apothecary are included in an entourage that could conceivably aid in the forthcoming attack; the apothecary holds an enema syringe, or clyster, as if to threaten his enemies with so potent a weapon.

34

The Dissolution; or The Alchymist Producing an Aetherial Representation

James Gillray (English, 1757–1815)

1796

Hand-colored etching

14⁵⁄₁₆ x 10³⁄₁₆" (36.4 x 25.9 cm) (plate)

17¹⁄₈ x 11⁹⁄₁₆" (43.5 x 29.4 cm) (sheet)

1988-102-93

Gillray's print was inspired by the power shown by Prime Minister William Pitt in dissolving Parliament and calling for new elections in May 1796. Pitt is portrayed as an alchemist, seated at a large retort in his laboratory, using the king's crown as a bellows, and surrounded by the symbols and apparatus of his arcane calling. The mortar at his feet holds Britannia's shield; bottles on the shelves are labeled "Oil of Influence," "Extract of British Blood," and "Spirit of Sal Machiavel[li]"; and he holds in his pocket a prescription for "Antidotus Republica." By representing the product of the distillation as Pitt enthroned as "Perpetual Dictator," Gillray is commenting on the prime minister's ability to fashion a Parliament according to his liking, which subsequent events would indeed prove to be the case.

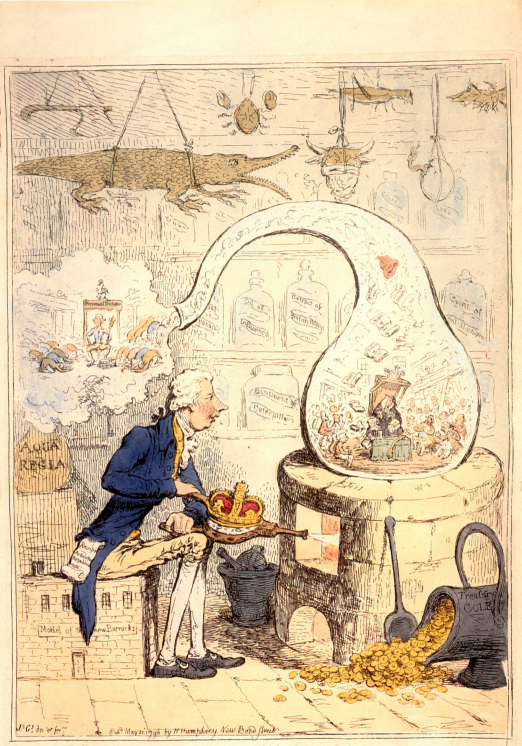

The DISSOLUTION, or The Alchymist producing an Aetherial Representation

35
Comfort to the Corns
James Gillray (English,
1757–1815)
1800
Hand-colored etching
9¹⁵/₁₆ x 7½" (25.3 x 19 cm) (sheet,
cropped within plate mark)
1988-102-90

The smile on the woman's face
points to the relief she has obtained
from the anguish caused by the
corns on the sole of her foot. Gillray
has made both her features and the
knife she uses disproportionately
large; even the cat watching the
operation seems out of scale.

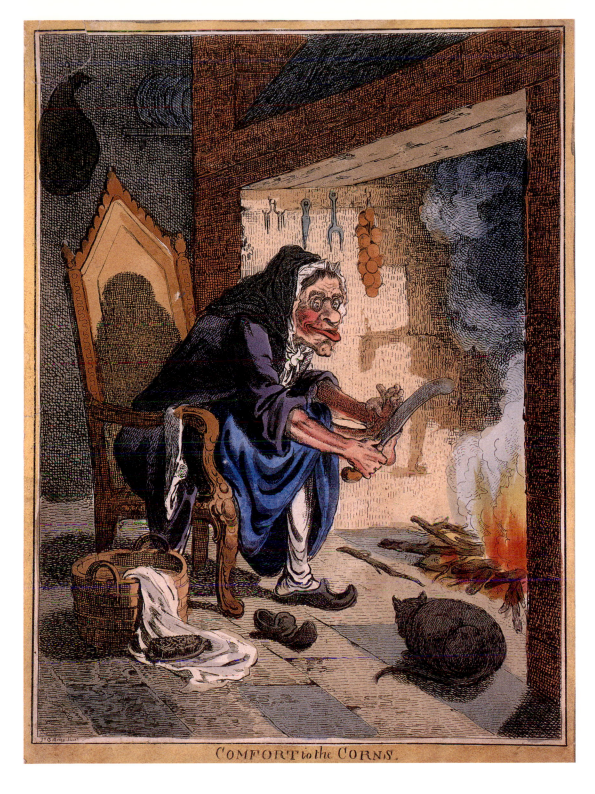

COMFORT to the CORNS.

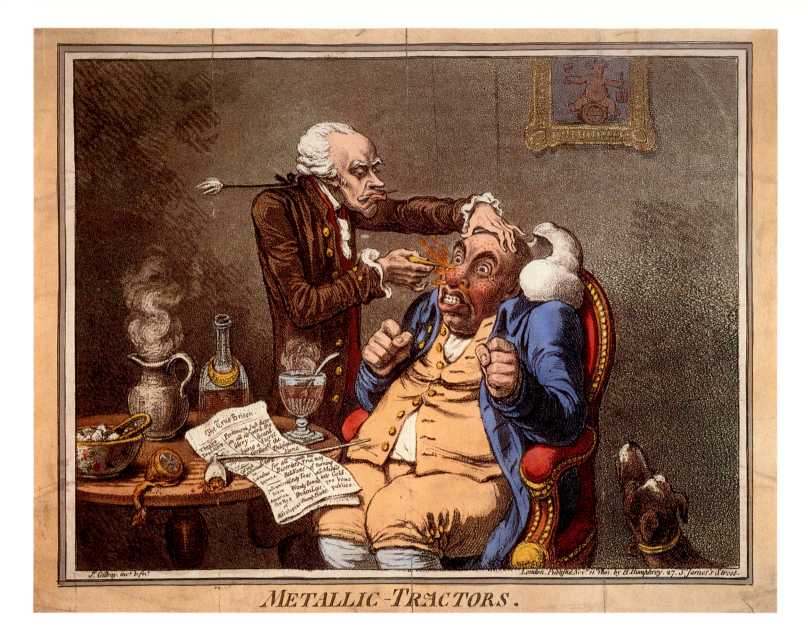

METALLIC-TRACTORS.

36

Metallic-Tractors
James Gillray (English,
1757–1815)
1801
Hand-colored etching and aquatint
9¾ x 12⁵/₁₆" (24.7 x 31.3 cm)
(sheet, cropped within plate mark)
1988-102-95

The operator applies metallic tractors to ease the pain of the carbun-
cles on the nose of his patient.
These brass and iron instruments,
which are about four inches long,
rounded at one end and flat and
slightly tapered at the other, had
been patented in 1796 by Elisha
Perkins, a Connecticut physician
who claimed his invention could
draw out disease by electrical force

(see also no. 6). The tractors were
taken to England by Perkins's son,
who marketed them successfully for
several years until they were proved
fraudulent. Gillray has here included
a squib in the newspaper on the
table boasting that the instruments
were "a certain Cure for all Disorders, Red Noses, Gouty Toes, Windy
Bowels, Broken Legs, Hump Backs."

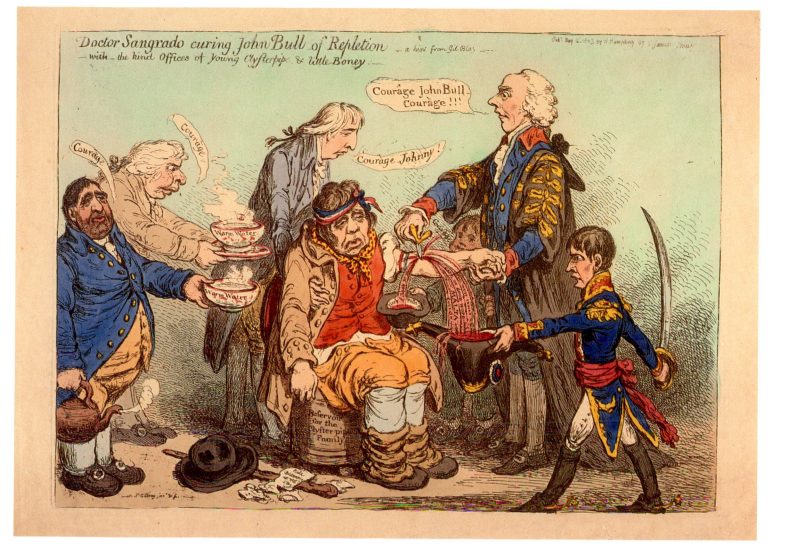

37

Doctor Sangrado Curing John Bull of Repletion with the Kind Offices of Young Clysterpipe & Little Boney
James Gillray (English,
1757–1815)
1803
Hand-colored etching
10³/₁₆ x 13¼" (25.9 x 33.6 cm)
(plate)
13¼ x 17¹¹/₁₆" (33.6 x 44.9 cm)
(sheet)
1988-102-94

In *L'Histoire de Gil Blas de Santillane*, an eighteenth-century novel by Alain René Lesage, Dr. Sangrado is a physician whose treatments are limited to bloodletting and drinking hot water. He was a well-known character to early nineteenth-century audiences, and his name itself came to be synonymous with *quack*. Gillray's parody uses the figure of Dr. Sangrado to complain

about the excessive taxation imposed by the government of Henry Addington in order to continue England's long war with France. An already weakened John Bull is being bled copiously as Napoleon holds out his hat to catch the spurting blood. Addington was frequently caricatured as an apothecary or, as here, a physician, largely because his father had been a doctor, and

Gillray and his contemporaries could not find a more appropriate symbol for so colorless a political figure (see also nos. 38, 39). In this print he is aided by other politicians—Charles James Fox; Robert Banks Jenkinson, Lord Hawkesbury; and the playwright Richard Brinsley Sheridan—two of whom hold bowls of warm water, one of Dr. Sangrado's favored remedies.

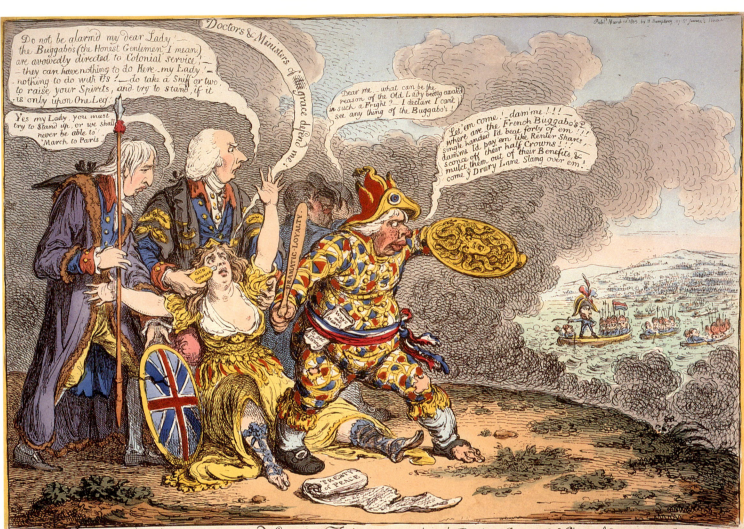

Physical Aid, — or — Britannia recover'd from a Trance; — also, the Patriotic Courage of Sherry Andrew, & a peep thro' the Fog —

38

Physical Aid, or Britannia Recover'd from a Trance
James Gillray (English, 1757–1815)
1803
Hand-colored etching
10⁷/₁₆ x 14⁵/₁₆" (26.5 x 36.3 cm) (plate)
10³/₄ x 14⁵/₈" (27.3 x 37.1 cm) (sheet)
1988-102-96

As the personification of England, Britannia appeared in political prints long before John Bull (see nos. 37, 45), and she was just as frequently attended by doctors when in distress. Here she is supported by Henry Addington, the prime minister, and Lord Hawkesbury, the foreign secretary, while the playwright-politician Richard Brinsley Sheridan (see nos. 37, 39) prepares to confront Napoleon and his armies, who are arriving from France. Addington offers the fainting Britannia a flask of gunpowder to inhale, but she rejects it, parodying Hamlet (1.4.39) in crying, "Doctors & Ministers of disgrace defend me!" Gillray crossed out the "dis," but clearly meant it to be read.

39
Confederated-Coalition; or The Giants Storming Heaven
James Gillray (English, 1757–1815)
1804
Hand-colored etching
17⅝ x 12¹⁵⁄₁₆" (44.7 x 32.8 cm)
(sheet, cropped within plate mark)
1988-102-91

The "Confederated-Coalition" is composed of those politicians, led by such men as Charles James Fox and William Pitt, who were united in their opposition to the ruling ministry in Great Britain in 1804. The focus of their attack is the prime minister, Henry Addington, who is caricatured as an apothecary wielding a large clyster as he defends the Treasury in the upper portion of the print (see nos. 37, 38).

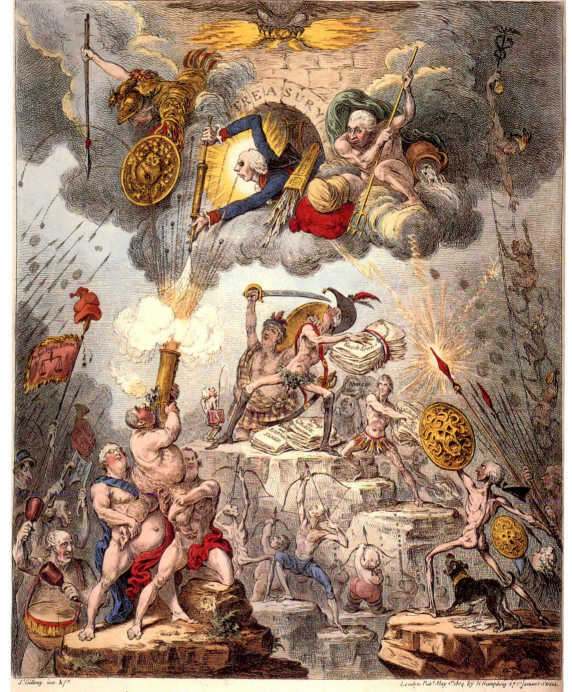

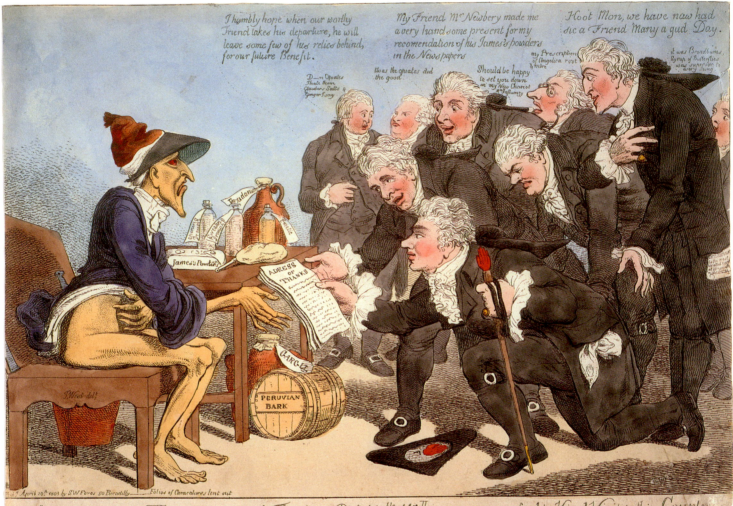

40
An Address of Thanks from the Faculty to the Right Hon[ora]ble Mr Influenzy for His Kind Visit to This Country
James West (English, n.d.)
1803
Hand-colored etching
9½ x 13⁵⁄₁₆″ (24.1 x 33.8 cm)
(sheet, cropped within plate mark)
1988-102-131

Doctors' fees have long been a frequent theme in medical satire, for no one wants to pay for illness and thus any expense can be deemed to be excessive. West's caricature shows a group of physicians who have been more than pleased to have benefited from an epidemic of influenza, and have thus come to pay homage to the disease for

increasing their incomes. Some of the medicines they have used, including a barrel of Peruvian bark (quinine) and bottle of gargle, lie under and on the table.

41

Dropsy Courting Consumption

Thomas Rowlandson (English,
1756–1827)

From "Tegg's Caricatures," no. 45

1810

Hand-colored etching

13¹¹⁄₁₆ x 9½" (34.8 x 24.1 cm)
(plate)

15¹⁵⁄₁₆ x 10⁷⁄₁₆" (40.5 x 26.5 cm)
(sheet)

1988-102-121

Rowlandson's obese man and emaciated woman represent the respective
ravages of edema and tuberculosis.
Both of them, as well as two figures,
one lean and the other fat, walking
arm-in-arm in the background, are
contrasted to a statue of Hercules,
symbolizing physical perfection,
placed in a nearby garden.

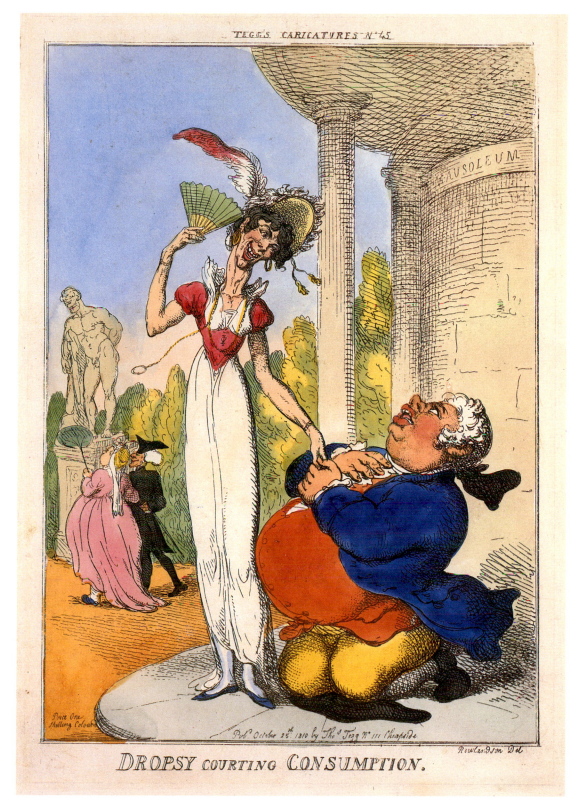

TEGG'S CARICATURES Nº 45

DROPSY COURTING CONSUMPTION.

42

Nursing the Spawn of a Tyrant, or Frenchmen Sick of the Breed

Thomas Rowlandson (English, 1756–1827)

1811

Hand-colored etching

13¹¹/₁₆ x 9¾" (34.8 x 24.8 cm) (plate)

15¹⁵/₁₆ x 10¼" (40.5 x 26 cm) (sheet)

1988-102-122

The Empress Marie Louise, the second wife of Napoleon, is appalled by the behavior of their son, who threatens her with a dagger; a bishop offers to calm the child with a goblet of "Composing Draught." The child's behavior and features, not surprisingly, resemble those of his father, who peers from behind a curtain. British artists lost no opportunity in mocking and deriding Napoleon in any way they could during the long course of the wars between Britain and France, and any aspect of his life, public or private, was considered a proper subject for caricature.

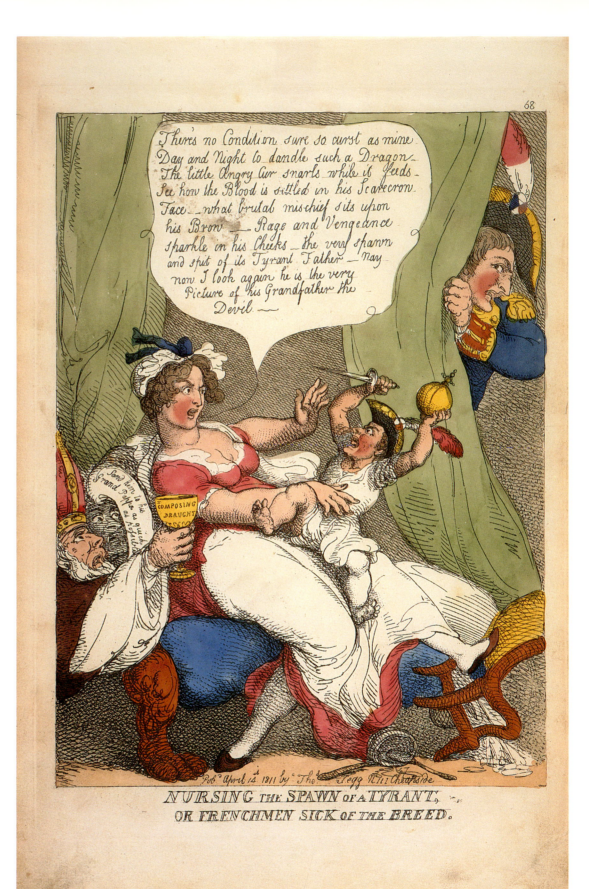

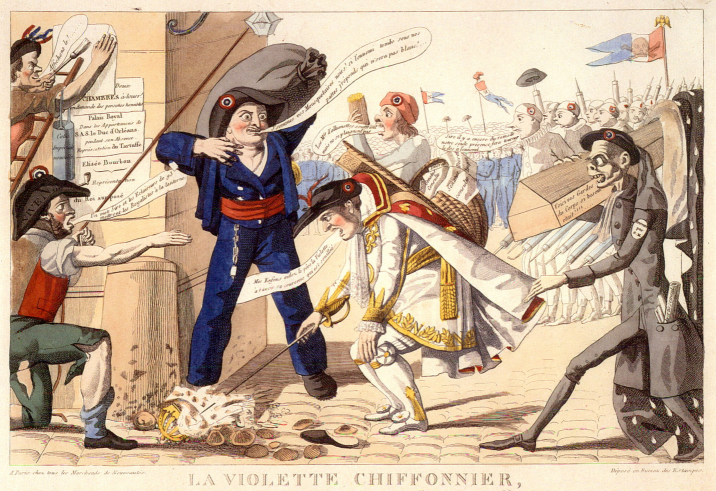

LA VIOLETTE CHIFFONNIER,
Cherchant sa couronne dans les ordures des faubourgs de Paris.

43
La Violette Chiffonnier (The Violet Ragpicker)
Anonymous, French
c. 1815
Hand-colored etching
9½ x 13¹/₁₆" (24.1 x 33.2 cm)
(sheet, cropped within plate mark)
1988-102-28

The French were not permitted to publish caricatures of Napoleon during his long reign, but after the emperor's exile to Elba in 1814, such satires began to appear in quantity. *La Violette Chiffonnier*, or *The Violet Ragpicker*, shows Napoleon, whose emblem was the violet flower, and a group of his supporters rummaging through trash heaps on the streets of Paris, looking for his tarnished crown. Instead of an honor guard of soldiers, the treasure seekers are attended by only a group of apothecaries, armed not with rifles but with clysters, their ever-present symbol in French political caricature.

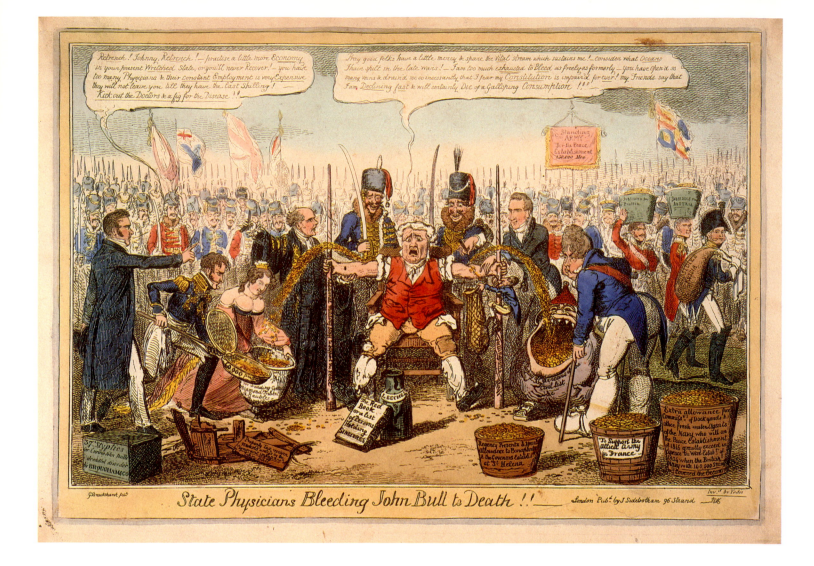

State Physicians Bleeding John Bull to Death !!

44

State Physicians Bleeding John Bull to Death!!

George Cruikshank (English, 1792–1878)

1816

Hand-colored etching

10⁵/₁₆ x 14¹³/₁₆" (26.2 x 37.6 cm) (plate)

11¹/₁₆ x 16¹⁵/₁₆" (28.1 x 43 cm) (sheet)

1988-102-65

Bleeding the patient has long been a worthy metaphor for excessive taxation (see no. 37). In this comprehensive attack on the possibility of increased taxes for military expenditures, John Bull is bled by two surgeons, Nicholas Vansittart, Chancellor of the Exchequer, and Robert Stewart, Viscount Castlereagh, the foreign secretary. The flow of gold guineas from his veins is copious, but as insurance, should the process not yield a sufficient amount, a jar of leeches is available. A gout-ridden Prince Regent, later King George IV, ruefully observes the proceedings.

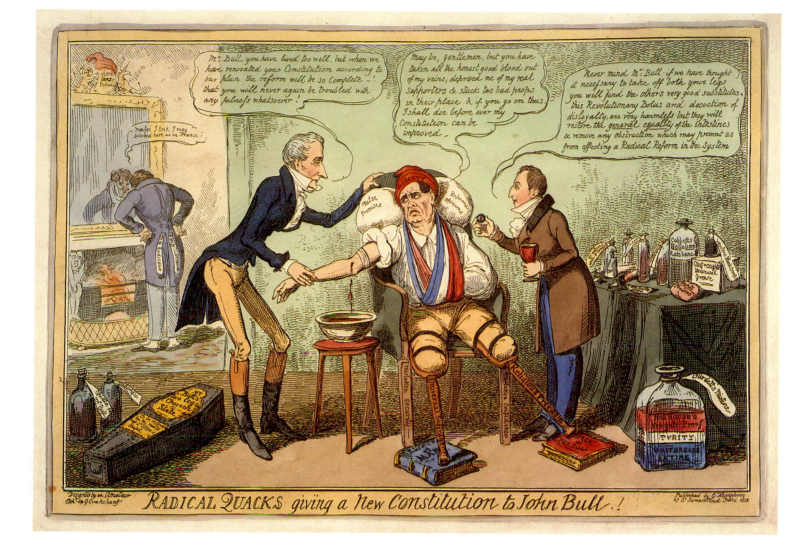

45
Radical Quacks Giving a New Constitution to John Bull!
George Cruikshank (English, 1792–1878)
1822
Hand-colored etching
9½ x 14³/₁₆″ (24.1 x 36 cm) (plate)
11¹⁵/₁₆ x 16¹³/₁₆″ (30.3 x 42.7 cm) (sheet)
1988-102-64

Cruikshank's print is representative of a common theme in political caricature: a nation, in this case England personified by John Bull, being treated by physicians (see nos. 37, 38, 44, 53). While the doctors offer medicines, surgery, and other medical procedures, their proposed solutions never seem to work. John Bull's doctors in this satire on pro- posed parliamentary reform are two radical members of Parliament from Westminster, Sir Francis Burdett and John Cam Hobhouse, Baron Broughton de Gyfford; their numer- ous remedies include bleeding, amputation, opiates, and a variety of eponymous potions.

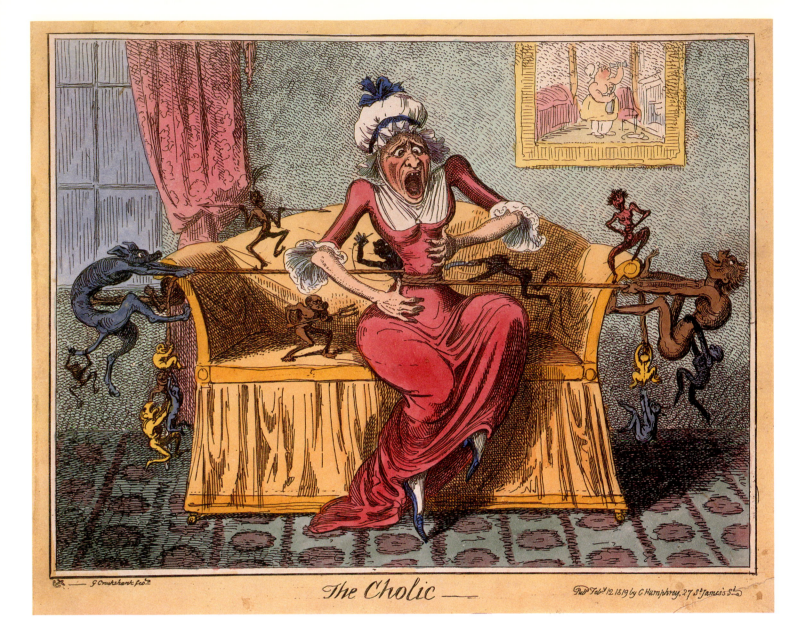

The Cholic —

46
The Cholic
George Cruikshank (English,
1792–1878)
1819
Hand-colored etching
8 1/16 x 10 1/16" (20.5 x 25.5 cm)
(sheet, cropped within plate mark)
1988-102-60

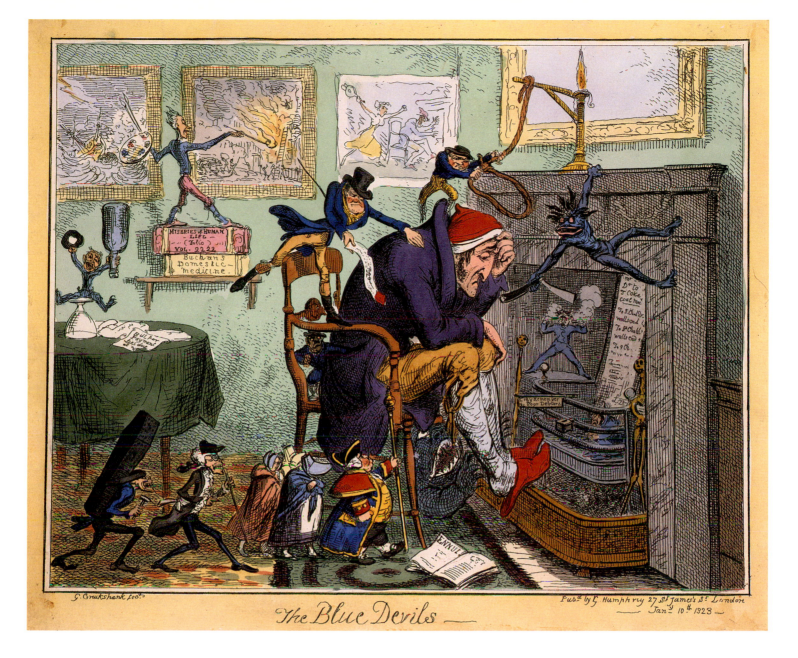

The Blue Devils —

47

The Blue Devils
George Cruikshank (English,
1792–1878)
1823
Hand-colored etching
8¼ x 10¹/₁₆" (21 x 25.5 cm) (sheet,
cropped within plate mark)
1988-102-59

Both *The Cholic* (no. 46) and *The Blue Devils* (no. 47) portray the horrors of illness. In the former, the vicious demons pulling on a taut rope wrapped around the woman's waist illustrate the acute paroxysmal abdominal pain associated with colic. As if the pulling were insufficient, others aid in the attack with spears and knives. *The Blue Devils* is no less severe in showing the torments of depression. Not only do the fiends assault the ill-fated victim, but the paintings on the wall, the titles of the books, the lists of debts to be paid, and the procession of a beadle, pregnant women, physician, and undertaker carrying a coffin also join in adding to the man's overall misery.

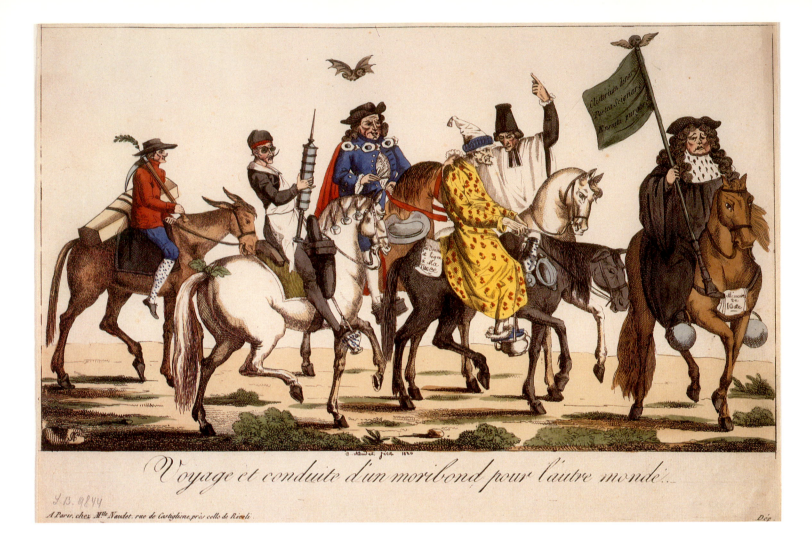

Voyage et conduite d'un moribond pour l'autre monde.

48

Voyage et conduite d'un moribond pour l'autre monde (Journey of a Dying Man to the Other World)
Caroline Naudet (French, 1775–1839)
1820
Hand-colored etching
9 x 13¼" (22.9 x 33.6 cm) (sheet, cropped within plate mark)
1988-102-116

A frequently encountered subject in French *imagerie populaire*, or popular prints (see no. 111), was the procession of the dying man accompanied on his voyage to the next world by his retinue of professional aides. In this early nineteenth-century version, the procession is led by a solemn physician, followed by a clergyman, surgeon, apothe-cary, and undertaker. The message on the physician's banner, "Cliste-rium donare, Postea seignare, Ensuita purgare" (To give a clyster, after that to bleed, finally to purge), echoes the treatment proposed for every disease by the doctors in Molière's satire of 1673, *Le Malade imaginaire* (see also no. 57).

49
Physic
Henry Heath (English, active
c. 1824–32)
1825
Hand-colored etching
12⁵⁄₁₆ x 8¹³⁄₁₆" (31.2 x 22.3 cm)
(sheet, cropped within plate mark)
1988-102-102

The cluttered counter in Heath's
pharmacy appears in sharp contrast
to the many handsome drug jars,
show bottles, and rows of attractively
labeled drawers. There is also a
contrast between the concerned
faces of the pharmacist and his
client, and the look of extreme
boredom shown by the apprentice,
contemplating his difficult and
lengthy task of manipulating an
oversize mortar and pestle. The
prepared prescriptions bear long
triangular labels (see no. 116),
a form still in use in Russia and
Scandinavia.

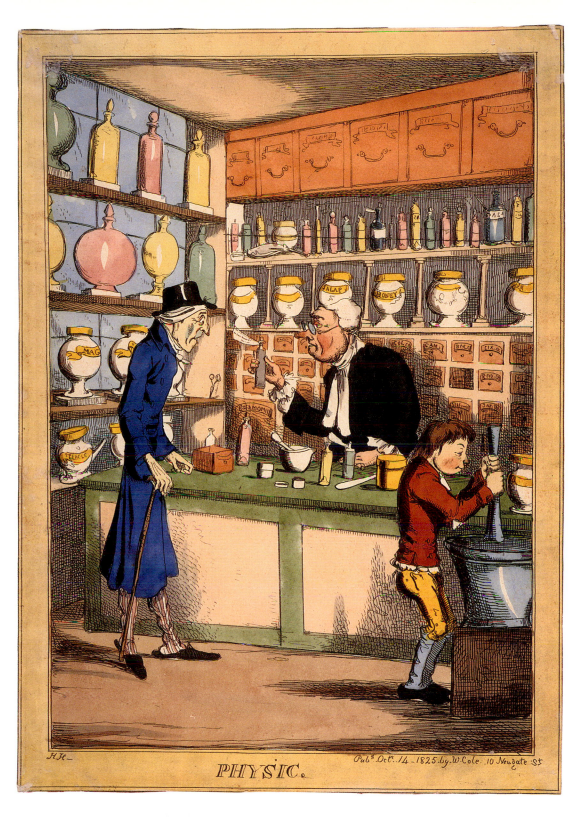

PHYSIC.

Pubᵈ Octʳ 14 1825 by W Cole 10 Newgate Sᵗ

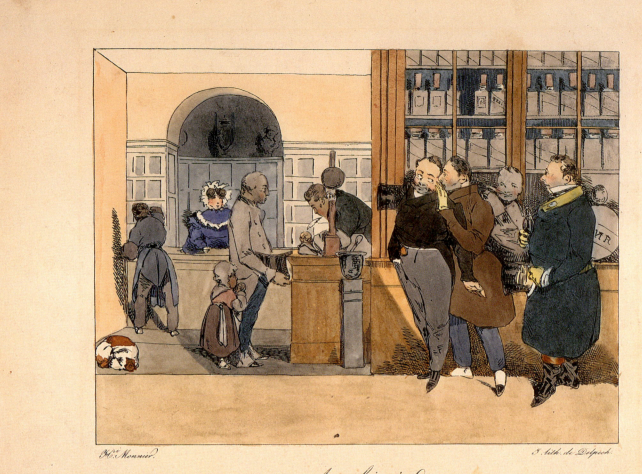

Hte Monnier.   Lith. de Delpech.

Apothicaire..

3.

50

Apothicaire (Apothecary)
Henry Monnier (French,
1805–1877)
late 1820s
Hand-colored lithograph
6⁵⁄₁₆ x 8³⁄₈″ (16 x 21.2 cm) (image)
9³⁄₄ x 12⁵⁄₁₆″ (24.8 x 31.3 cm)
(sheet)
1988-102-115

Fashionably dressed clients are
attended in an elegant pharmacy,
with rows of bottles behind glass
doors and a large show bottle on a
counter nearby. While others at the
counter look on, one man tries to
give another sufficient courage to
overcome his embarrassment in
approaching the pharmacist for his
request.

51

Keeping the Child Quiet: Scene at Batts Hotel—No. 2
William Heath (English, 1795–1840)
1829
Hand-colored etching
14⁵⁄₁₆ x 9¹⁵⁄₁₆" (36.4 x 25.2 cm)
(sheet, cropped within plate mark)
1988-102-103

Daniel O'Connell, the Irish statesman, was elected a member of Parliament in 1828, but there was considerable question over whether he, as a Catholic, could properly take his seat. He is the sick child in the print; three parliamentary colleagues—Henry Peter Brougham, Sir James Macintosh, and Sir Francis Burdett—supporters of proposed reforms to admit O'Connell, are charged with keeping him tranquil until this decision can be made. O'Connell holds a rattle labeled "MP," and both a bottle of soothing syrup and a steaming bowl of gruel are necessary to maintain his serenity.

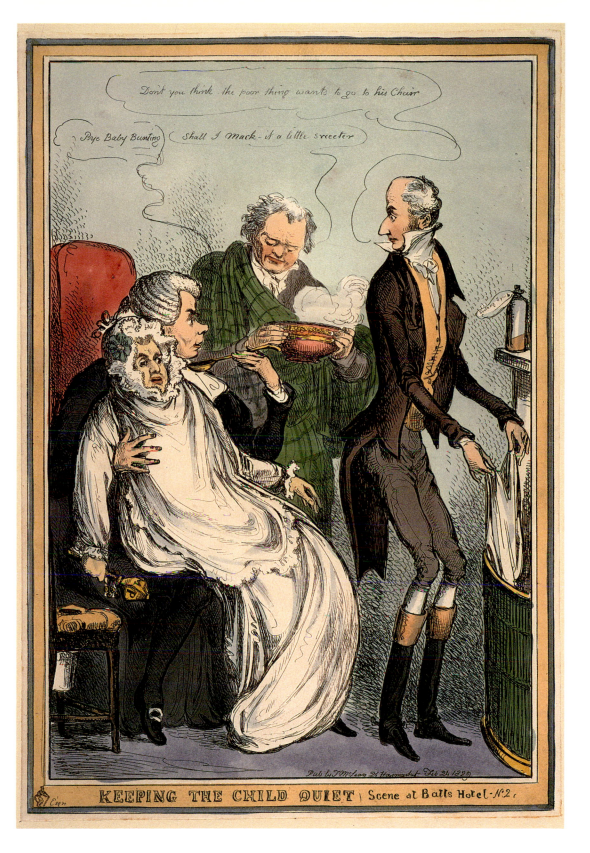

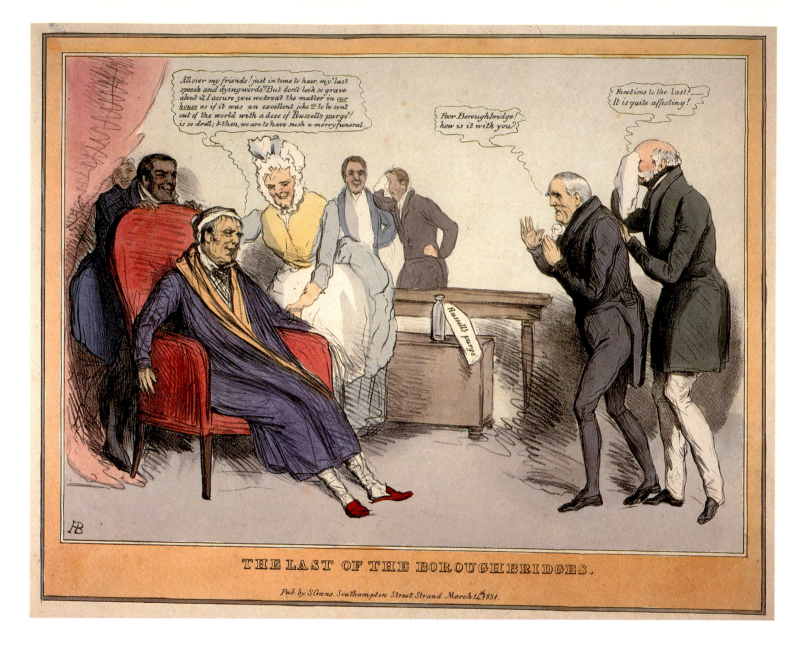

THE LAST OF THE BOROUGHBRIDGES.

Pub. by. S. Gans. Southampton Street. Strand March 1st 1831.

52

The Last of the Boroughbridges
John Doyle (English, 1797–1868)
1831
Hand-colored lithograph
10³⁄₈ x 13⁵⁄₁₆" (26.4 x 33.8 cm)
(image)
11⁹⁄₁₆ x 15" (29.4 x 38.1 cm)
(sheet)
1988-102-75

Sir Charles Wetherell, member of Parliament for Boroughbridge, steadfastly opposed Sir John Russell's proposal for parliamentary reform that would eliminate Wetherell's seat. The bottle of "Russell's purge," which has caused his forthcoming demise, rests on a table nearby, and his friends and political allies look on with various reactions.

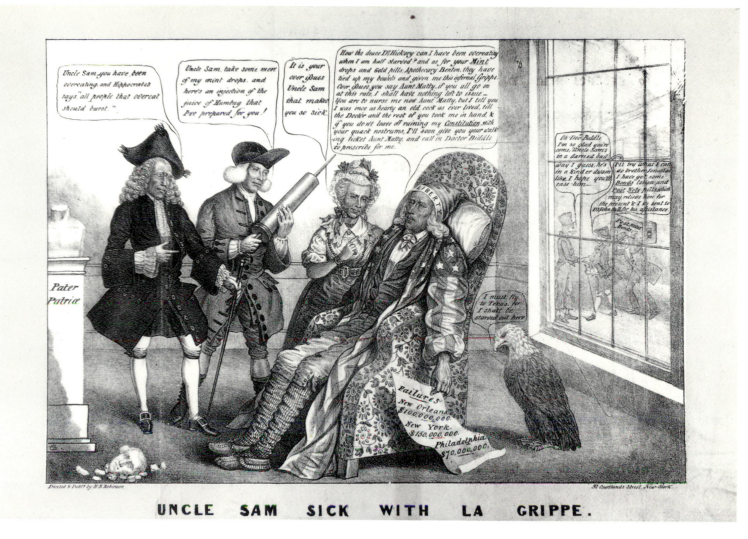

UNCLE SAM SICK WITH LA GRIPPE.

53

Uncle Sam Sick with La Grippe
Edward Williams Clay (American, 1799–1837)
1834
Lithograph
11 x 15¹⁵/₁₆" (27.9 x 40.5 cm) (image)
13 x 18¹³/₁₆" (33 x 47.7 cm) (sheet)
1988-102-120

The "grippe" from which Uncle Sam is suffering is the economic crisis precipitated by President Andrew Jackson's veto of the bill to recharter the Bank of the United States and his subsequent demand that only hard currency be used in payment for federal lands. Those ministering to the sick nation include the president as the physician; Jackson's vice-president and eventual successor Martin Van Buren as the nurse; and his political ally Senator Thomas Hart Benton as the apothecary holding a clyster. Jackson's lack of success in improving Uncle Sam's condition had led to the call for another doctor, and Nicholas Biddle, former head of the national bank, can be seen arriving. Biddle is greeted by Brother Jonathan, who was, like Uncle Sam, a frequent symbol of the United States in the nineteenth century; the print is unique in showing both figures simultaneously.

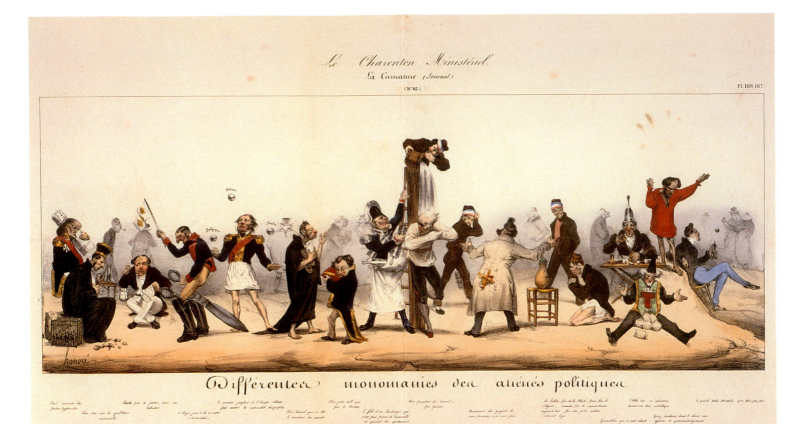

54

Le Charenton ministériel (The Ministries of Charenton)
Honoré Daumier (French, 1808–1879)
From *La Caricature*, no. 83 (May 31, 1832), pls. 166–67
Hand-colored lithograph
7¹¹/₁₆ x 20″ (19.5 x 50.8 cm) (image)
13³/₈ x 21³/₈″ (33.9 x 54.3 cm) (sheet)
1988-102-70

Charles Philipon's weekly journal *La Caricature* kept up a relentless attack on the government of Louis-Philippe, the "Citizen King," using whatever means possible to satirize those in power (see also nos. 55–57). In this print the inmates of the mental asylum at Charenton, each engaged in some deranged act, are either members of Louis-Philippe's government or one of its supporters.

Daumier chose this setting because of press reports of symptoms of madness toward the end of the life of Prime Minister Casimir Périer. Here the central figure, shown at a makeshift shower with three enema syringes, is Georges Mouton, comte de Lobau, a general under Napoleon who later became commander of the National Guard in Paris. In quelling

Bonapartist riots near the Place Vendôme, Lobau had resorted to high-pressure hoses; the caricaturists seized on the event to make the enema syringe his symbol (see also nos. 55–57). Daumier describes him in the text as the "son of a baker who became prince of the triple clyster pipe and apothecary general."

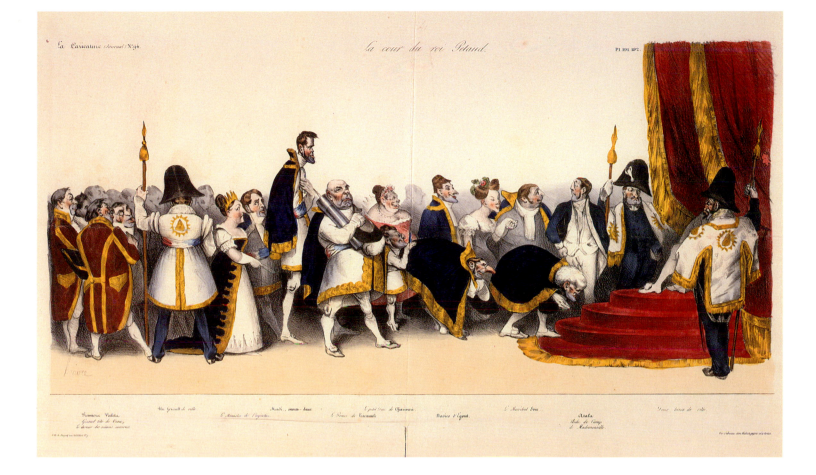

55

La Cour du roi Pétaud (The Court of King Pétaud)
Honoré Daumier (French, 1808–1879)
From *La Caricature*, no. 94 (August 23, 1832), pls. 191–92
Hand-colored lithograph
10¹¹/₁₆ x 20⅛" (27.1 x 51.1 cm) (image)
13⁵/₁₆ x 21³/₁₆" (33.8 x 53.8 cm) (sheet)
1988-102-69

In another of Daumier's attacks on Louis-Philippe (see also nos. 54, 56, 57), government dignitaries, dressed in their finest costumes, have come to pay homage to the Citizen King. In the center of the group is the bald, heavy-jowled, scowling loyalist, the comte de Lobau, holding a clyster as though it were a military weapon. Daumier labels him "Le Prince de Tricanule," an allusion to this instrument (*la canule*).

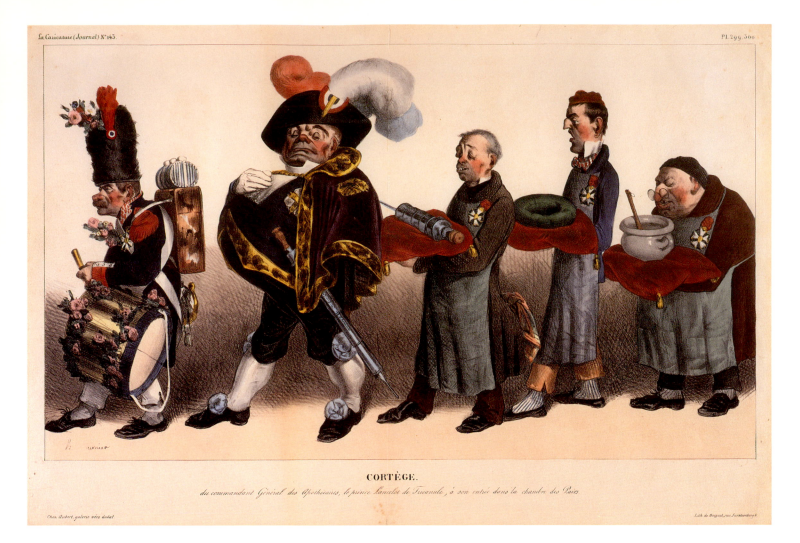

CORTÈGE.

du commandant Général des Apothicaires, le prince Lancelot de Tricanule, à son entrée dans la chambre des Pairs.

56

Cortege

Honoré Daumier (French, 1808–1879)

From *La Caricature*, no. 143 (August 1, 1833), pls. 299–300

Hand-colored lithograph

11⅝ x 19⅞" (29.5 x 50.4 cm) (image)

14 x 21¼" (35.6 x 54 cm) (sheet)

Lent by William H. Helfand

Even a minor event such as the elevation of the comte de Lobau to the peerage in 1833 was sufficient for Daumier's inspired mockery of the government of Louis-Philippe (see also nos. 54, 55, 57). Here he shows Lobau as the "commandant Général des Apothicaires, le prince Lancelot [a play on the phrase *lance l'eau*, or throwing water] de Tricanule," marching at the head of a procession. His attendants carry his various badges of office: a clyster, a cushion, and a chamber pot.

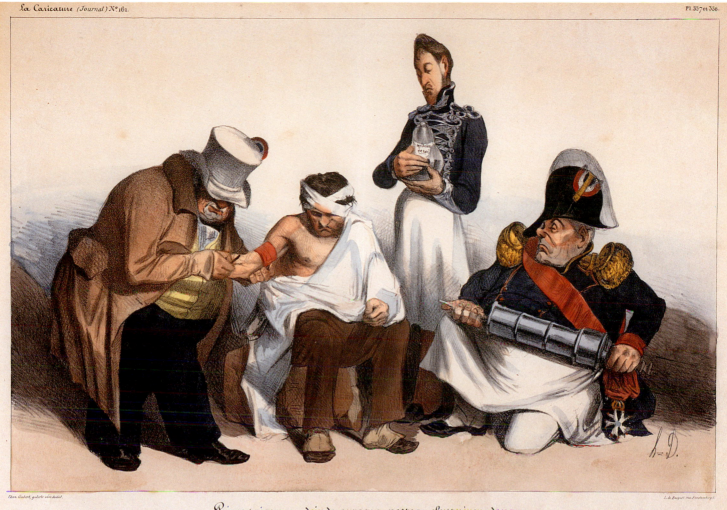

La Caricature (Journal) N°.161.

Pl. 337 et 338.

Chez Aubert, galerie véro dodal.

L. de Becquet, rue Furstenberg 6.

Primo saignare, deinde purgare, postea clysterium donare.

D'abord saigner, ensuite purger, postérieurement seringuer.

(Quelques personnes traduisent Deinde par le mot diarde, mais c'est un latin de Cuisine.)

57

Primo saignare, deinde purgare, postea clysterium donare (First to Bleed, Then to Purge, Finally to Give a Clyster)
Honoré Daumier (French, 1808–1879)
From *La Caricature*, no. 161 (December 5, 1833), pls. 337–38
Hand-colored lithograph
11⁹⁄₁₆ x 17³⁄₈" (29.4 x 44.1 cm) (image)
14 x 20⁷⁄₈" (35.6 x 53 cm) (sheet)
Lent by William H. Helfand

In October 1833 a mailman named Wernet was run over by a coach just as Louis-Philippe and his family passed by. The king, who as a youth had medical training during an apprenticeship at the Hôtel-Dieu in Paris, came to the aid of the mail-man, and his gesture, as would be expected, was well received by the public. Daumier has seized on this event as yet another occasion to attack the regime (see also nos. 54–56), presenting Wernet as the down-trodden French people, bled by the king's lancet, clystered by the comte de Lobau, and drugged by the bottle of the "médecine Le roi" that is held by Louis-Philippe's son, the duc d'Orléans. (The treatment itself recalls the one proposed in Molière's satirical *Le Malade imaginaire* [see no. 48].) The name of the medicine is a play on words that alludes to both the king and a well-known laxative, the Purgatif Le Roy.

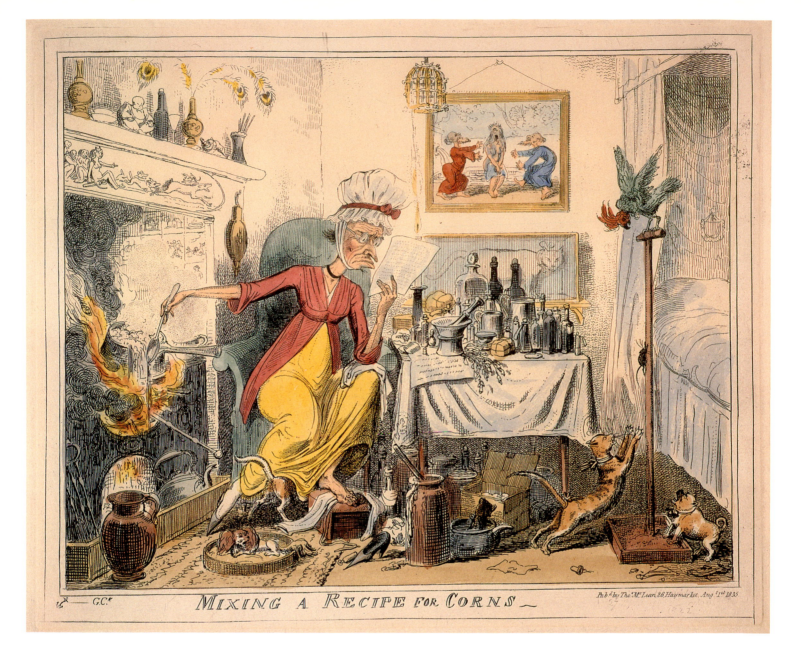

MIXING A RECIPE FOR CORNS—

58

Mixing a Recipe for Corns
George Cruikshank (English, 1792–1878)
1835
Hand-colored etching
8³/₁₆ x 9³/₄″ (20.8 x 24.8 cm) (plate)
8¹/₂ x 10⁵/₁₆″ (21.6 x 26.1 cm) (sheet)
1988-102-61

The table is not large enough to hold all the ingredients necessary for a recipe for her corns that the grotesque woman is preparing, and bottles and jars have been spread out on the floor as well. The woman is oblivious to the dogs, cats, and other animals running loose, and even ignores the flame from a candle that has set fire to her bonnet. Her mixture has alarmingly begun to boil over, but she remains equally unaffected by the forthcoming disaster.

59
Souvenirs du choléra-morbus
(Memories of Cholera)
Honoré Daumier (French,
1808–1879)
From François Fabre, *Némésis
médicale illustrée: Recueil de
satires* (Brussels: Bruylant-
Christophe et Compagnie, 1841),
p. 41
Wood engraving
10 x 6½ x 1″ (25.4 x 16.5 x 2.5 cm)
(bound)
1988-102-71

The Paris physician François Fabre
published his series of satirical
verses on medical practices in two
volumes in Paris in 1840, followed
by a one-volume edition in Brussels
the next year. The twenty-five chap-
ters on subjects such as phrenology,
homeopathy, hospitals, clinics,
pharmacists, and charlatans criti-
cized various aspects of medicine
and defended the necessity for
freedom in medical education. They
were accompanied by thirty wood
engravings, mainly caricatures, by
Daumier. Not all were designed to be
humorous; this print from the chap-
ter on cholera, for example, shows a
dead man lying in the street, another
being carried to a waiting hearse,
and a funeral procession passing in
the background.

SOUVENIRS DU CHOLÉRA-MORBUS. 41

Emprisonner sans fin dans un étroit *cordon*
Le coursier indompté qui court à l'abandon,
Et séquestrant Paris d'une immense ruine,
Purger au lazaret la vengeance divine !
Hélas ! de quel espoir se berce l'insensé !
A travers lazarets et cordons élancé,
Transporté par les vents sur l'aile des nuages,
Le monstre tôt ou tard nous gardait ses ravages.
Paris épouvanté l'aperçut un matin ;

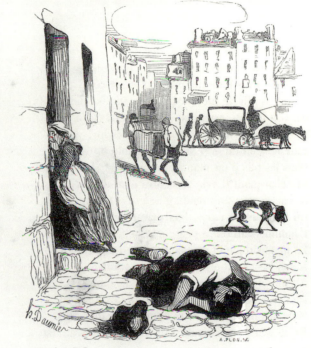

1ʳᵉ SÉRIE. E. B.   6

60
Medical Confessions of Medical Murder
Anonymous, English
c. 1840
Wood engraving
17³/₈ x 22⁵/₁₆" (44.1 x 56.6 cm) (sheet)
1988-102-14

Advertisements for Morison's Vegetable Pills, composed of strong cathartic ingredients, often went to extremes in rejecting the orthodox approach to medicine in favor of the Morisonian belief that all diseases arose from impurities in the blood that the vegetable pills could cure (see also no. 61). Here twelve medical scenes illustrate statements from physicians, often taken out of context, that denounce unnecessary surgery, excessive prescribing of potent medicines, ineffectiveness of hospitals, and other baneful practices. Several prominent members of the medical profession are quoted, including the anatomist Matthew Baillie, the surgeon Anthony Carlisle, and James Johnson, physician to King William IV. Even Shakespeare contributes to the general condemnation of conventional treatments with his "Throw physic to the dogs, I'll none of it" (*Macbeth* 5.3.40).

61
Singular Effects of the Universal Vegetable Pills on a Green Grocer! A Fact!
C. J. Grant (English, n.d.)
From "Grant's Oddities," no. 8
1841
Hand-colored lithograph
10³/₄ x 9⁷/₈" (27.3 x 25 cm) (image)
16¹³/₁₆ x 11¹⁵/₁₆" (42.7 x 30.3 cm) (sheet)
1988-102-100

The promotion of Morison's Vegetable Pills in the 1830s and 1840s was not only ubiquitous but also excessive, promising cures for a wide spectrum of ailments, including tuberculosis, jaundice, and tic douloureux (see also no. 60). Not surprisingly, such immoderate claims provoked critical and satirical reaction. Grant's print shows the frightening—but humorous—side effects produced when a green grocer was caught in the rain after having taken "132 Boxes of Vegetable Pills"; since this event occurred on April 1, however, it cannot be meant to be taken too seriously.

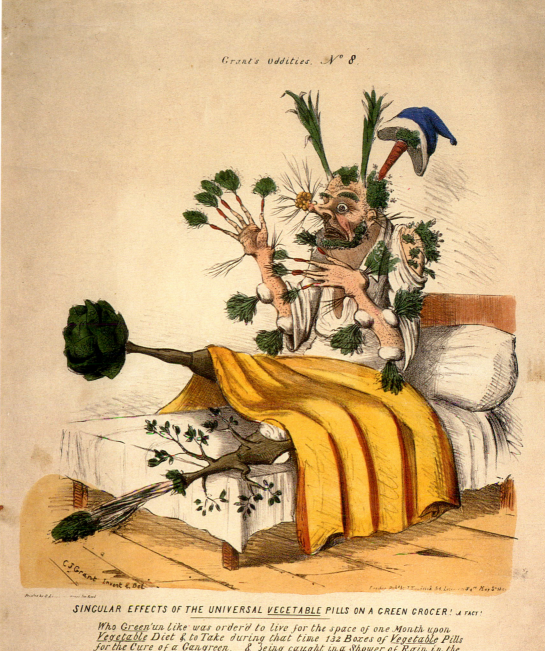

Grant's Oddities. N° 8.

CJ Grant Invent & Del.

SINGULAR EFFECTS OF THE UNIVERSAL VEGETABLE PILLS ON A GREEN GROCER! A FACT!

Who Green'un like was order'd to live for the space of one Month upon
Vegetable Diet & to Take during that time 132 Boxes of Vegetable Pills
for the Cure of a Gangreen. & Being caught in a Shower of Rain in the
Green Fields in the evening of the 1ˢᵗ of April last, was put to Bed 'midst
Shooting pains, & in the Morning presented the above Phenomenon of a
Moving Kitchen Garden !!!

Query —   Is he not one of the Productive Classes.

62
Situation intéressante (A Financially Interesting Situation)
André Gill (professional name of Louis Alexandre Gosset de Guines, French, 1840–1885)
Cover of *L'Eclipse*, 5th year, no. 196 (July 28, 1872)
Hand-colored relief print
13^{15}/$_{16}$ x 11^{5}/$_{16}$" (35.4 x 28.7 cm) (image)
18^{7}/$_{8}$ x 13^{5}/$_{16}$" (47.9 x 33.8 cm) (sheet)
1988-102-87

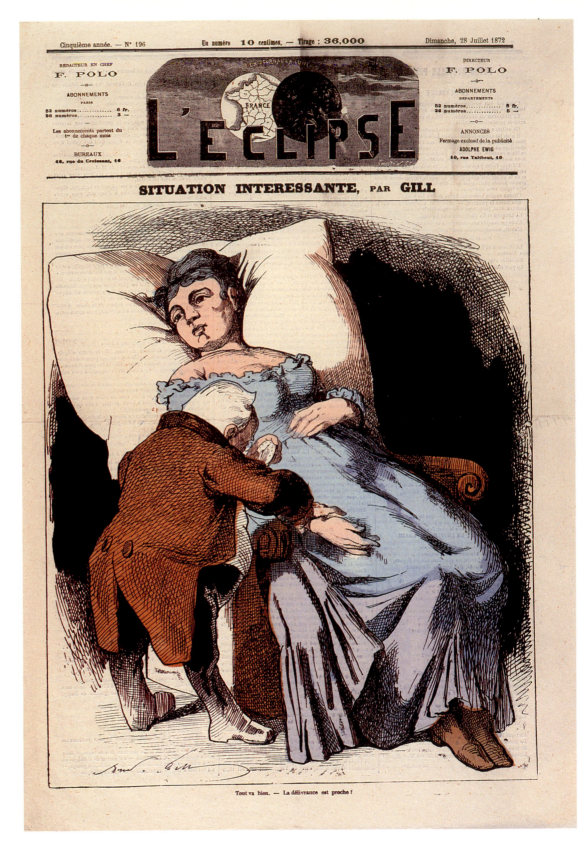

63
La Délivrance (The Delivery)
André Gill (professional name of
Louis Alexandre Gosset de Guines,
French, 1840–1885)
Cover of *L'Eclipse*, 5th year, no. 197
(August 4, 1872)
Hand-colored relief print
14 x 11¾" (35.5 x 29.8 cm)
(image)
19¼ x 12⅞" (48.9 x 32.7 cm)
(sheet)
1988-102-84

The obstetrician in both of these
caricatures is Louis Adolphe Thiers,
the president of the French Third
Republic. Gill uses the metaphor of
childbirth to comment on Thiers's
negotiations for the loan that France
sorely needed to pay reparations to
Germany in the aftermath of the
disastrous Franco-Prussian War of
1870–71. In *A Financially Interesting Situation* (no. 62), he is ready to
deliver France's child, and the
caption, "The delivery is close,"
suggests that the funds will soon be
forthcoming. In Gill's second caricature (no. 63), published one week
later, the loan has been secured, and
Thiers proudly exhibits the newborn
for all to see. As a result of the
censor's potent control, clouds cover
all but the feet of four figures at the
bottom of this print. Gill had
intended them to represent Napoleon III and leaders of the fallen
Bonapartist, Bourbon, and Orléanist
factions, each of which had objected
to such an early settlement of the
indemnity.

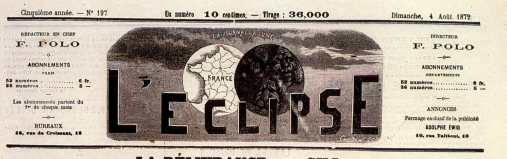

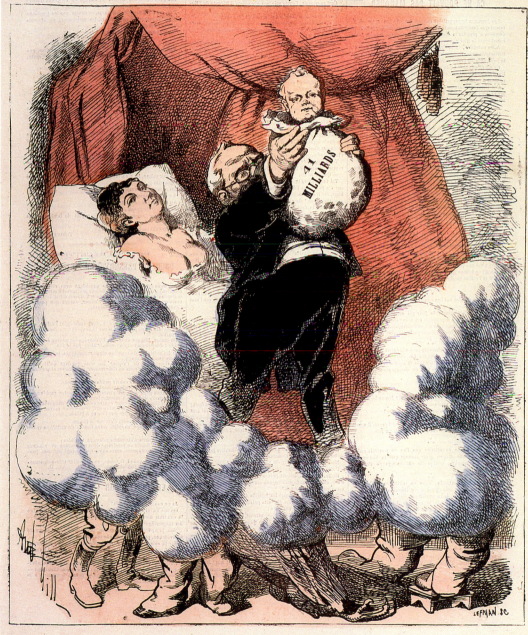

64

Le Dr Ricord
André Gill (professional name of
Louis Alexandre Gosset de Guines,
French, 1840–1885)
Cover of *La Lune*, 3rd year, no. 85
(October 20, 1867)
Hand-colored relief print
19¹⁄₈ x 13⁷⁄₁₆″ (48.6 x 34.1 cm)
(sheet)
1988-102-85

The physician Philippe Ricord, who
was born of French parents in Balti-
more, devoted his long career to the
understanding and treatment of
venereal disease. Among other
contributions, he was the first to
show that syphilis and gonorrhea
were independent conditions, and
he also clearly delineated the various
stages and types of syphilis. Here
Ricord holds a surgical knife as his
attribute.

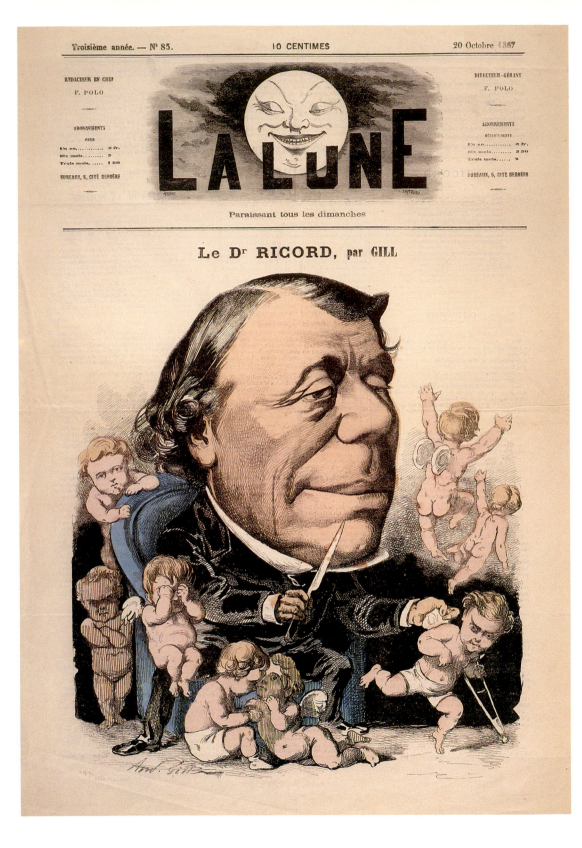

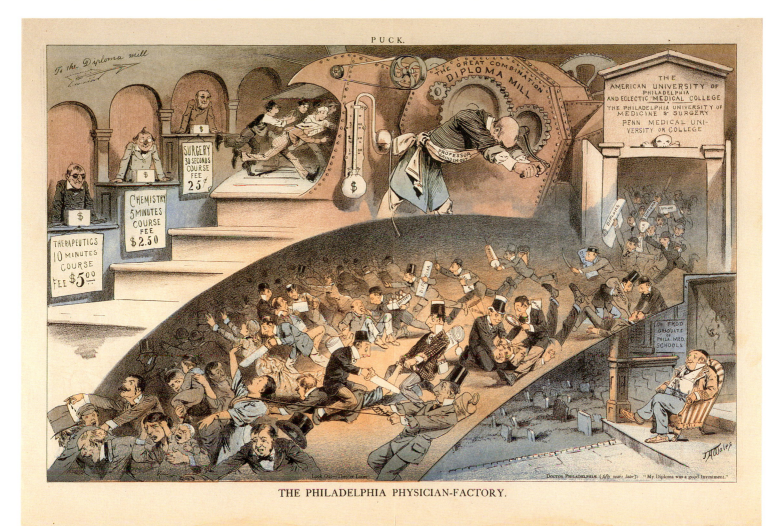

THE PHILADELPHIA PHYSICIAN-FACTORY.

65

The Philadelphia Physician-Factory
James Albert Wales (American, 1852–1886)
From *Puck*, vol. 7, no. 162 (April 14, 1880), pp. 94–95
Color lithograph
11³⁄₄ x 18⁹⁄₁₆″ (29.8 x 47.1 cm) (image)
13¹⁵⁄₁₆ x 20¹¹⁄₁₆″ (35.4 x 52.5 cm) (sheet)
1988-102-130

The appalling lack of standards in medical education in the latter part of the nineteenth century, and in particular the excessive number of "diploma mills," prompted this outraged comment in *Puck*. Philadelphia, despite its many legitimate medical schools, including that of the University of Pennsylvania, the oldest in the United States, was used as the focus for Wales's merciless attack. While the university itself is not mentioned, variations on its name are listed on the portal of the building from which the newly graduated physicians, their diplomas held high, emerge as the public is warned, "Look Out—They're Loose!"

66

Better Not Vaccinate Than Vaccinate with Impure Virus

Joseph Keppler (American, born Austria, 1838–1894)

From *Puck*, vol. 7, no. 171 (June 16, 1880), p. 276

Color lithograph

11⁹⁄₁₆ x 8⅝" (29.3 x 21.9 cm) (image)

13⅜ x 9⅞" (34 x 25.1 cm) (sheet)

1988-102-109

Controversy over the smallpox vaccination began almost immediately upon the announcement of Edward Jenner's discovery in 1798, for the concept of administering a totally foreign agent into the bloodstream aroused a great deal of apprehension. The cow carrying a container of "impure virus" echoed the public's long-standing concern over vaccine quality, and demands arose for assurance that the lymph would be completely free of bacteria and viruses that might cause syphilis, tuberculosis, erysipelas, and other dire infections.

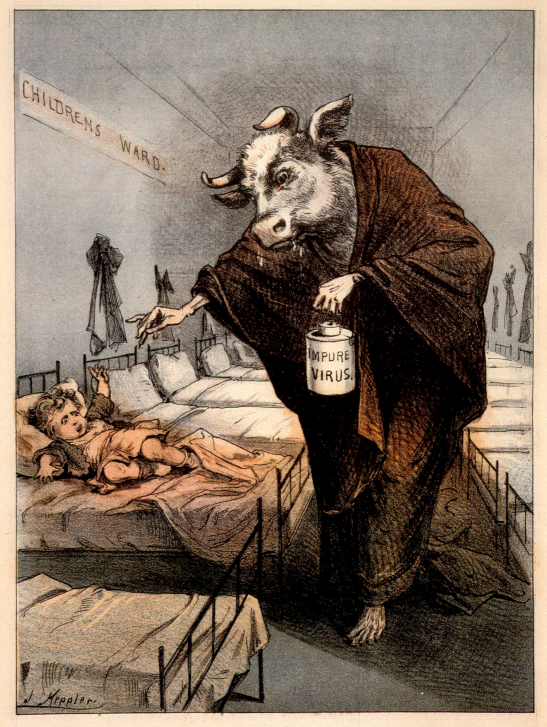

BETTER NOT VACCINATE THAN VACCINATE WITH IMPURE VIRUS.

67
**Esculape: La Truffe au médecin et
la drogue au client (Aesculapius:
Truffles for the Doctor and Drugs for
the Patient)**
Charles Maurin (French,
1854–1914)
1892
Lithograph
11¹⁵/₁₆ x 9⁷/₈" (30.3 x 25 cm)
(sheet)
1988-102-113

Maurin's lithograph may have been
designed as a cover for a menu.
Aesculapius, the Roman god of
medicine, who is identified by the
staff on his back, offers a bowl of
truffles to the doctor and a bottle of
medicine to his patient. There is a
marked contrast between the figures: The physician, holding a long
bone as his walking stick, is formally
dressed and totally absorbed in the
food awaiting him rather than in his
patient, who is drawn only partially
covered but equally preoccupied.
Maurin's depiction of the male
doctor's insensitivity may have been
his comment on the medical profession's attitude toward women.

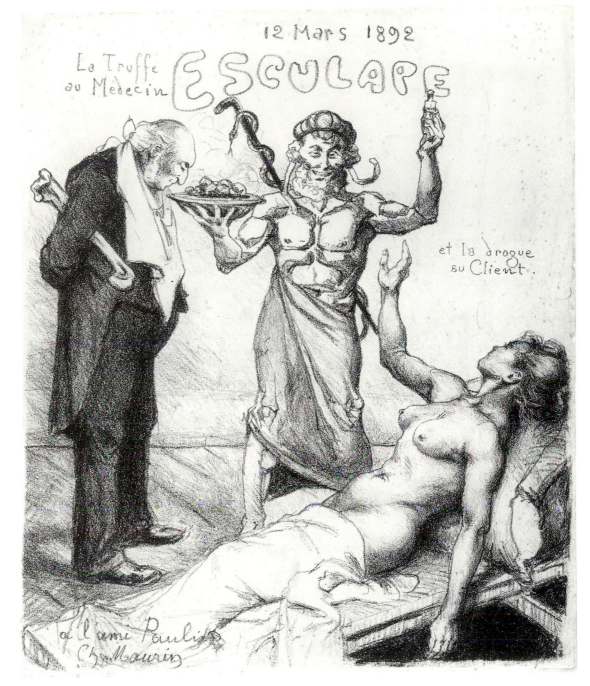

68
Les Médecins (The Doctors)
Jules-Abel Faivre (French,
1867–1945)
Cover of *L'Assiette au beurre*, no. 51
(March 22, 1902)
Lithograph
12½ x 9⅜" (31.8 x 23.8 cm)
(sheet)
1988-102-76

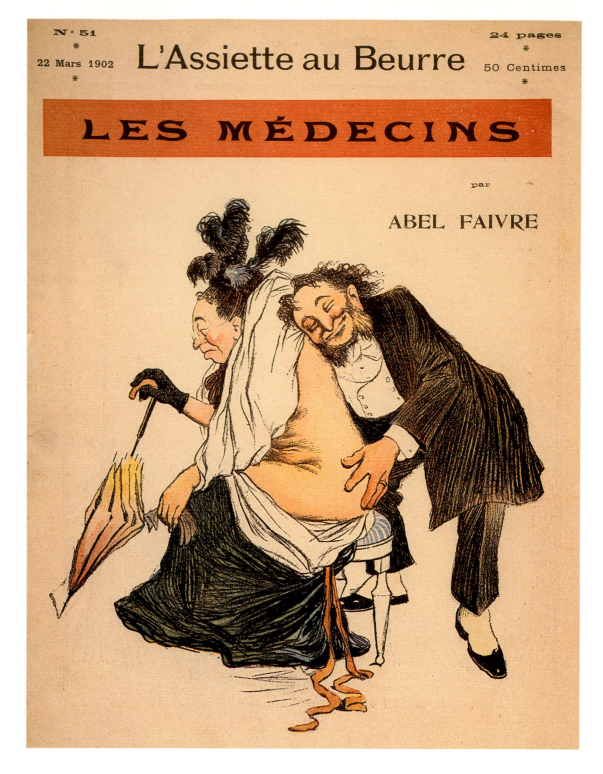

69
Les Pharmaciens (The Pharmacists)
Démétrius Emmanuel Galanis
(French, born Greece, 1882–1966)
Cover of *L'Assiette au beurre*, no.
107 (April 18, 1903)
Lithograph
12½ x 9⅜" (31.8 x 23.8 cm)
(sheet)
1988-102-80

L'Assiette au beurre appeared
weekly from 1901 to 1912, and
later briefly in 1921–22. Each issue
contained a series of caricatures
devoted to a single theme, with
many illustrated by one artist.
Faivre, the son of a physician, produced twenty-four caricatures of
physicians in one issue in 1902 (no.
68), and Galanis published an equal
number in a publication devoted to
pharmacists one year later (no. 69).
The majority of the illustrations in
both are mild caricatures, but several of those by Faivre on surgical
mishaps, such as the surgeon who
must stop halfway through an unsuc-
cessful amputation, are devastating.

N° 107
18 Avril 1903

L'Assiette au Beurre

40
Centimes

LES PHARMACIENS
Par GALANIS

L'HOMME A TOUT FAIRE

Il peut extraire les fibrômes,
Il fait au besoin un trépan,
Scientifique sacripant,
Véritable Apache à diplômes.

Il se fait prince de la Sonde
Ou bien extirpeur de chicots,
Il est — « Maman-tire-le-monde »
Son quartier l'égale à Charcot.

Le voici médecin pour dogues
Au besoin masseur de tibias
Ou bien dévideur de tœnias
Mais, avant tout, il vend ses drogues.

Il prétend dompter la hernie
Ou faire repousser le poil,
Ou bien vous donner du géni
En vous électrisant la moëlle

Dieu du ciel ou du Walhalla,
Apaisez nos justes alarmes,
Car on est nu, seul et sans armes,
Vis-à-vis de ce bougre-là.

JEHAN RICTUS

70
Dame Jacinthe
Théophile-Alexandre Steinlen
(French, 1859–1923)
From "Chansons d'Aïeules"
("Ancestral Ballads")
1900
Lithograph
9¹/₁₆ x 7¹/₁₆" (23 x 17.9 cm)
(image)
13¹¹/₁₆ x 10¹¹/₁₆" (34.8 x 27.1 cm)
(sheet)
1988-102-126

The suggestion that male physicians
might have an interest in their
female patients for other than medical reasons has led to many satirical
drawings. Steinlen's lithograph
shows a leering doctor attending his
fashionable patient in a scene that
looks as if it might have taken place
in the eighteenth century, more than
one hundred years before the print
was made.

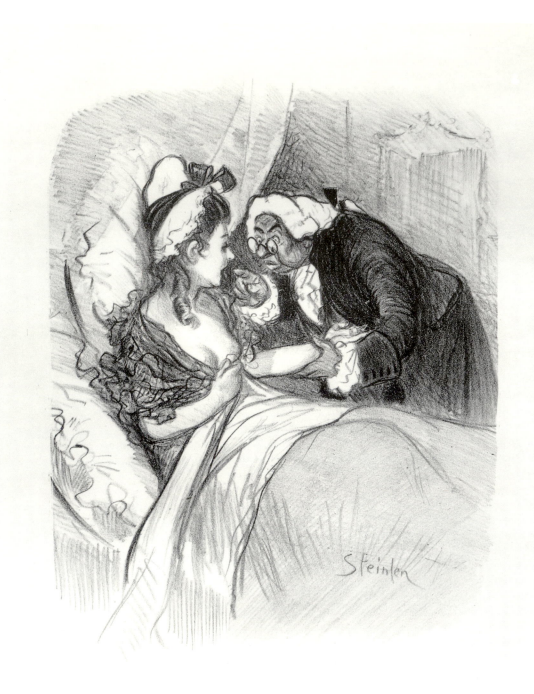

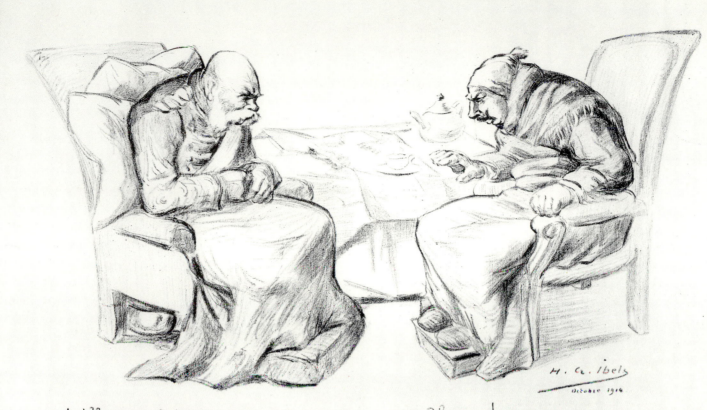

Guillaume: Qu'est ce que nous prenons pour mon Rhume!

71
Guillaume: Qu'est ce que nous prenons pour mon Rhume! (Wilhelm: What Shall We Do for My Cold!)
Henri-Gabriel Ibels (French, 1867–1936)
1914
Lithograph
17³/₄ x 25⁵/₁₆" (45 x 64.3 cm) (sheet)
1988-102-106

French perceptions of the troubles facing the alliance between Germany and Austria at the onset of World War I are symbolized by the two men bundled in blankets: Kaiser Wilhelm II of Germany and the Emperor Franz Josef I of Austria. Ibels shows these leaders as old and feeble, an assessment that was not, however, shared by their military forces.

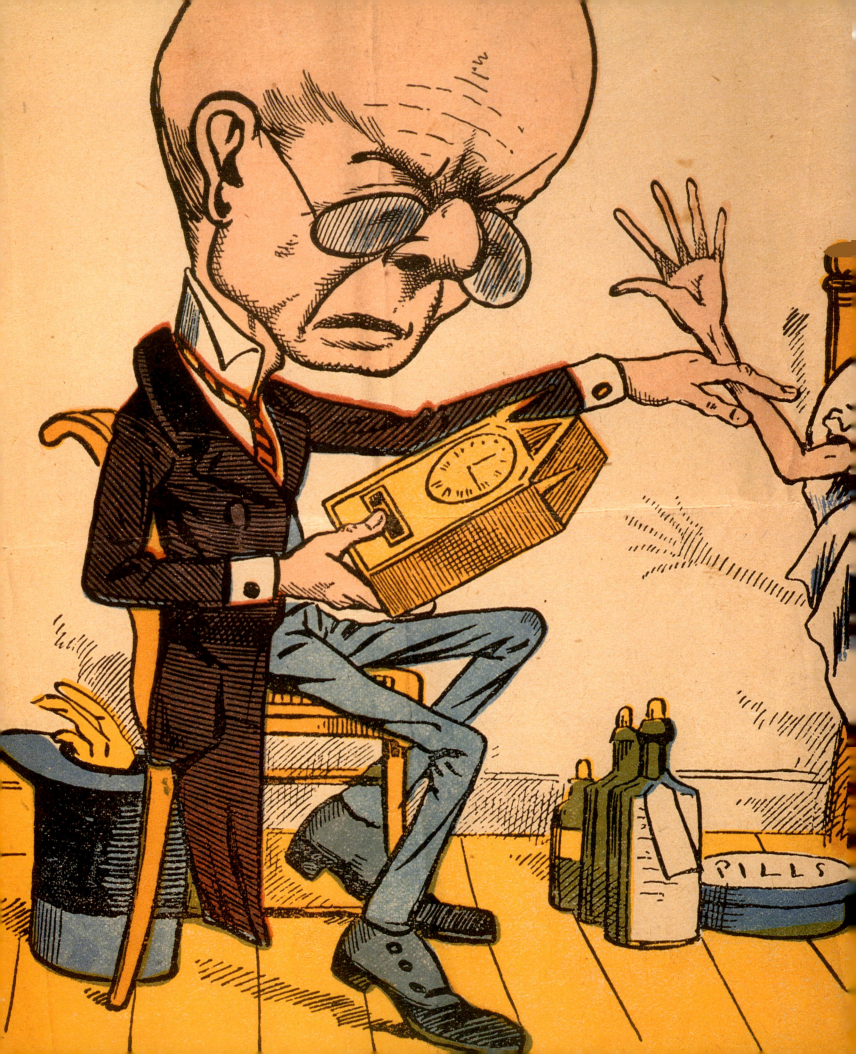

The Art of Medical Ephemera

Maurice Rickards

Detail of the *Quack Doctor* valentine (no. 117)

The term *ephemera* has been defined as "the minor transient documents of everyday life."[1] The word derives from the Greek *epi* (about) and *hemera* (a day). It refers (as it does when applied to the mayfly) to something lasting hardly more than a single day. In terms of printed papers the word covers all those passing fragments, important today and rubbish tomorrow, that so often find their way at the end of the day to the wastebin.

Tickets, flyers, notices, labels, stationery, packaging, advertisements—these and scores of other transients serve their little function and then are gone. Their rescue, conservation, and study have in recent years become a major research activity, for although they are conceived as throwaways, they may now survive as lasting items of evidence. As with all such memorabilia, they carry the unmistakable marks of the period that brought them into being. In their style, their subject matter, and the attitudes and mores they reflect, they are a vital part of the social history record.

Medical ephemera is no exception. In collections, public and private, all over the world, printed throwaways are being gathered—physicians' stationery, pharmacists' labels, trade cards, flyers, packaging, prescriptions, and calling cards—the evidential research material of the history of healing.

New collections are being formed; existing ones are being searched. Specialized holdings, like that in the Wellcome Institute Library in London, continue to yield new finds, as do general ones like the New-York Historical Society's Bella C. Landauer Collection. Sometimes discoveries come by chance: *objets trouvés* in cellar or attic, accidental heirlooms in family papers, time-capsule finds in abandoned stores. At other times they appear in dealers' lists or as lots in auction catalogues. Wherever they emerge, the ephemerist is there to round them up as part of the general record.

Ephemera may be sorted, broadly speaking, under two main heads: *category* and *theme*. *Category* refers to the general function of the item; *theme*

1. Membership application form, Ephemera Society, London, 1978.

relates to its subject matter. Typical categories are tickets, billheads, trade cards, and packaging; themes may include subjects such as fashion, football, drama, or dogs. Some collections are organized only by category, others only by theme, and still others confusingly by both.

In medical ephemera, categories—flyers, trade cards, prescriptions, and the like—are fairly clear-cut. Themes are wide-ranging: from vaccination to battlefield surgery, obstetrics to quackery. The structure of a collection is shaped in part by the availability of the material and in part by the expertise and aspirations of the collector. Some collections grow from accidental accumulations, such as the long-forgotten printer's specimen file or the bundle of family papers; others from an *ab initio* research decision, perhaps a desire to gather evidence of a certain social history trend or the development of an aspect of printing or graphic design.

However triggered, by accident or intention, the collection is an instrument rather than a mere possession. It is for study as well as admiration. It is, fundamentally, for use as *evidence*. Like all such evidence, medical ephemera illuminates the general as well as the particular. In its typography, its printing technology, its design, and its editorial assumptions, it reflects its period. But above all it conveys the history of medicine and its impact on society.

In the present exhibition, with its scatter of themes and categories, we observe the highs and lows, the fads and fancies, of medical and pharmaceutical practice. Here, in the Belgian village of Grammont in the mid-nineteenth century, we have Dr. de Cock (no. 76) with his newly coined water-sweating treatment (surely not far removed from the classic Turkish bath, but better value under the title of *établissement hydrosudopathique*). Here too are Pike's Toothache Drops (no. 100), dedicated not only to curing "the most violent and protracted toothache" but to saving the teeth. With this product medical science has moved on from the healing properties of water and sweat to those of morphine and opium.

Less specific are the ingredients in the English Female Bitters (no. 83), a concoction good for everything from premenstrual tension to prolapsus of the uterus. (Bitters of all kinds were popular among both sexes in the latter part of the nineteenth century, largely for their alcohol content.) Nichols' remedy (no. 98) cites "elixir," Peruvian bark, and protoxide of iron as its ingredients, extending their virtues to cover not only dyspepsia, indigestion, malarial fevers, general debility, loss of appetite, nervous prostration, and headache but, as a final safeguard, "hypochondria &c."

Medical ephemera also includes much peripheral — as opposed to promotional — material. Although no less historically significant, this category includes such items as medical lecture admission tickets, surgeons' certificates of competence, hospital rules and regulations, and out-patients' admission cards. These too are redolent of their period. A typical item, from about 1843, sets out the conditions governing patients' entry into the London Hospital: "Patients to provide themselves with a Quart Bottle, Gallipot and Phial. . . . no person . . . in a state of confirmed consumption, or deemed by the Physicians or Surgeons incurable . . . [is] admissible into the Hospital. . . . Presents of old Linen, large Quantities of which are used for Dressings and Bandages, will be thankfully received."[2]

Other peripheral ephemera includes such pieces as bookplates, illustrated stationery, sheet music covers, bookmarks, valentines, postcards, street-collection emblems, and charity stamps—all potential bearers of medical or pharmaceutical reference. Typical are the quack doctor satirical valentine (no. 117), an example of a genre popular on both sides of the Atlantic, and the series of music covers, chiefly British (nos. 119–24), dismissing the medical profession, the patient, and pills and plasters at large. Also among the humorous peripherals is a multitude of postcards, prints, and other items known as *imagerie populaire* (see nos. 110, 111),[3] in which doctor and patient alike are lampooned. (Humor, we may speculate, is in this context a function of bravado, a gesture of defiance at the machinations of the gods.)

In a class of their own are bookplates, a category well known for its personal eccentricity and in the medical field no less so (nos. 125–28). Here too we see, as in medical ephemera at large, a due scattering of classic attributes of the profession: the alembic, the mortar and pestle, and the ubiquitous syringe, or clyster, which had run riot as an irreverent symbol in the nineteenth century (see no. 128; see also nos. 73, 74, 77–79, 111, 112, 116).

It must be said that opinions differ as to the admissibility of the bookplate to the classification "ephemera." Firmly pasted in its allotted book, its role may be thought to be something less than transient, but it may well be argued (and often is) that the bookplate, *before* it is pasted, is as ephemeral as any bus ticket. The debate, however, continues.

Of all categories of medical ephemera, peripheral or promotional, by far the most prolific in numbers is the trade card. As its preponderant showing in this selection indicates, this humble item has a special place in the attentions of the ephemerist, collector and curator alike, and its survival in quantity makes it possibly the most accessible of all these transient forms of evidence.

I t was in America, particularly in the latter part of the nineteenth century, that the trade card had its day. For various reasons, this colorful item swept the nation, becoming even in its own time a talking point and universal album filler. The popular American trade card of the 1880s and 1890s had antecedents in the seventeenth and eighteenth centuries, when Europe's tradesmen were first beginning to find their feet. Printed from hand-engraved copperplates, these early promotional pieces gave customers the basics: the name and address of the business, the line of goods or services, and occasionally an image or two to catch the eye. They also did service as unofficial billheads. With the later addition of the phrase "Bought of," the billhead proper emerged. This was in turn to bring forth a further derivative: today's letterhead.

2. From the Petition to the House-Committee of the London Hospital, Ephemera Collection of the Foundation for Ephemera Studies, London.

3. This term, here used generically, is more specifically applied to the products of the Pellerin press at Epinal, France. See Leonard Marcus, ed., *An Epinal Album: Popular Prints from Nineteenth-Century France* (Boston, 1984).

At first the "card" was printed on paper. It was much later, when it had become general practice to print the images on card, that the term *trade card* came into use. The word was applied in retrospect even to the earlier paper versions, and is thus used in our own times. Ambrose Heal, in his *London Tradesmen's Cards of the XVIII Century*, makes the point that these early examples "were not cards, but sheets of paper ranging up to folio size." Writing in the mid-1920s, when the terminology was still fluid, he cites the naming options for this category of ephemera as tradesmen's bills, shopkeepers' bills, tradesmen's cards "—or the shorter form, 'Trade Cards.' "[4] He settles broadly for the shorter form (although retaining the longer one in the book's title).

The eighteenth-century trade card was a creation of some elegance—often, it may be said, a work of art. In Britain we find specimens by William Hogarth and Francesco Bartolozzi. Hogarth designed over a dozen trade cards, among them one for himself as an engraver and another for his sisters Mary and Ann, who kept a "frock-shop."[5] Bartolozzi did one for a London drawing master — "T. Sandby Junr. St. Georges Row, Oxford Street"—that listed his "Terms of teaching."[6]

Early American examples include designs by Paul Revere for the Boston store of Joseph Webb (1765) and for Isaac Greenwood, ivory turner, also of Boston (c. 1770). Another Boston card, designed by Nathaniel Hurd in 1774, advertises "Drugs & Medicines, Chymical & Galenical," that were sold by Philip Godfrid Kaft "at the Sign of the Lyon & Mortar in Salem."[7]

The Hurd card is among the first American medical trade cards. As with the work of many colonial engravers, it partakes of the conventions of some of its London counterparts, in this case including the hanging shop sign by which the druggist was identified.

The shop sign was a major feature of the early trade card. In London the heavy swinging board, on which the sign had first appeared, was banned in the 1760s as a public danger. The boards were ordered to be taken down and fixed flat against the shop fronts. This ruling was unpopular with tradesmen, however, who had relied on these images to help patrons locate their shops; they forthwith reproduced their signs on their trade cards, often including detailed directions for finding the place. In an era before street numbering came into general use, these instructions had to be specific, sometimes even elaborate: "Mary & Ann Hogarth . . . Removed to ye King's Arms joyning to ye Little Britain-gate near Long Walk," and "Gabriel Douce at ye Lamb & Black Spread Eagle next door to the Golden Goate in New Round Court in ye Strand."[8]

No less evocative of the period are the trades and occupations the cards portray. Heal's study discloses, among many designations, purveyor of asses' milk, bow and arrow maker, "Bugg Destroyer to His Majesty," chimney sweep, corn cutter, dancing master, lamplighter, and ratcatcher and sow gelder. The medical trades advertised included chemists, apothecaries, druggists, dentists, oculists, surgeons, surgical instrument makers, truss makers, cuppers, dog doctors, and skeleton sellers.[9]

4. Ambrose Heal, *London Tradesmen's Cards of the XVIII Century: An Account of Their Origin and Use* (1925; reprint, New York, 1968), p. 1.

5. Ibid., pls. XXX, XXXIV.

6. Ibid., pl. XXVII.

7. See American Antiquarian Society, Worcester, *A Society's Chief Joys: An Exhibition from the Collections of the American Antiquarian Society* (Worcester, 1969), p. 134, no. 268; pp. 114–15, no. 228.

8. Heal, *London Tradesmen's Cards*, pl. XXXIV.

9. Ibid., pp. 16, 36, 38–62, 90.

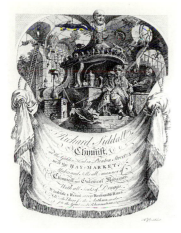

Fig. 1
Trade card for Richard Siddall
English, c. 1780
Engraving, 10 x 7" (25.4 x 17.8 cm)
Trustees of the British Library, London

Among the most splendid of all early medical ephemera is the trade card of Richard Siddall, maker and seller of "Chymical and Galenical Medicines," including the "Elixir for the Asthma, as also for the Gout and Rheumatism" (fig. 1). In this card we have the epitome of eighteenth-century up-market quackery—a composite of magic and spells, lizard and herb, phial and furnace—all the paraphernalia of the successful "Chymist." The design is remarkable not only for its multidisciplinary view of therapy but for its aesthetic appeal. Here in classic form is that most finely poised of images, a work of "commercial" art. Both Siddall and his engraver—one "R Clee"— demonstrate an early grasp of a medium that has come to rule our lives. Commercial art, and certainly that portion of it as expressed in promotional medical ephemera, may be said to start with this image. With this truly illustrious beginning, how far had this branch of graphic art gone in a hundred years, when the hand-printed black-and-white engraving had given way to the mass-produced, multicolored lithograph?

The color lithography process revolutionized pictorial printing.[10] Based on Aloys Senefelder's discovery of lithography in the 1790s, the technique allowed the superimposition of separate color images to build up as one brilliantly colorful "superimage." Each color was printed from an individual lithographic stone, sometimes a dozen or more in succession, each skillfully hand-prepared to contribute its own subtle effect in the final picture.

Progressively mechanized, the process developed hand in hand with the nineteenth century's mass-market society. By the time Louis Prang brought color lithography to the fore in America in the 1860s, mass production and mass marketing were hitting their stride. Like every other industry, the medical and pharmaceutical field was quick to exploit this marvelous new medium. The color lithographed trade card, in parallel with a plethora of greeting cards, calendars, and other novelties, moved into a position of dominance among printed ephemera, where it was to stay for thirty or forty years. By the 1880s the American color lithographed card had assumed the role of a New World institution. It appeared in countless millions, with a high proportion dedicated to the greater glory of pills, potions, and lotions.

As with its European counterparts, the American trade card was printed either as a "stock" card, on which the trader's name and message could be imprinted (nos. 103, 105), or as a "dedicated" design, custom-made to the advertiser's special needs (see nos. 83, 85, 92, 95). Either way, a popular gambit was the series, in which the purchaser was induced to acquire a complete set of cards, in the process becoming a regular customer. Receiving the cards separately over the counter or as giveaways packed in with the product, the addicted shopper soon became a collector. The principle was to be developed later in the cigarette card and, in America, the chewing gum card.

Both in America and Europe, the stock card had certain hazards, not least of which was the use of the irrelevant or inapposite image. Bright's Kidney Beans (no. 80), for example, had only the most tenuous link with the

10. For a brief outline of this and other printing processes, see Maurice Rickards, *Collecting Printed Ephemera* (Oxford, 1988), pp. 82–102.

clam, or for that matter the bathing girl, used to advertise the product, and the actresses on the Hop Pill cards (no. 89) could surely have had no notion of the "Headache, Nervousness, Dyspepsia, Liver Complaints and Constipation" that the medicine claimed to cure. Even a dedicated series of cards could run into trouble. As the well-meaning series for Cognet shows (no. 81), no promotional message is a match for outright horror, even in the sacred name of martyrology.

Considered as a work of art, the position of the medical trade card remains debatable. As with all promotional printed ephemera, while there is implicit acceptance of the need for graphic expertise, it is mostly a matter of good fortune as to who provides it. It must be said that few pieces of ephemera remotely approach the standard of the Richard Siddall card, and indeed it is only in a minority of cases that there are signs in that direction.

We may pick out a few splendors among the present selection. The "Aesthetic" figures advertising Star Cough Drops (no. 103) have a certain graphic authority, as do the Fernet-Branca set pieces (no. 86). The latter are typical of Italy's turn-of-the-century, neoclassical, all-purpose promotional images, with the product painted in—often at odds with perspective. Undoubted stars are the flower series for Cognet medicines (no. 82), unsigned and unblushing derivatives of the style of Alphonse Mucha, messages of hope from Paris to the cough-wracked Spanish. Here, each in a few square centimeters, are minor treasures, evidence at once for the medical historian, the printing specialist, the art historian, and the social history analyst.

But whatever our individual value judgments, however adequate or otherwise the items in this exhibition may have been in their time, and however effectively they serve as historical evidence, they remain as witnesses, worthy of our attention, care, and conservation. It is in collections like this one—and in institutions like the Philadelphia Museum of Art—that they find security and survival.

72
Trade Card for
Arnold, Chemist & Druggist
English, Norwich, late nineteenth
century
Engraving
3⁵/₈ x 2⁵/₁₆″ (9.2 x 5.8 cm)
1989-69-54

73
Trade Card for
**S. Moss, Druggist, Operative &
Experimental Chymist**
English, late nineteenth century
Engraving
3³/₁₆ x 4¹⁵/₁₆″ (8.1 x 12.5 cm)
(plate)
5 x 8⁷/₈″ (12.7 x 22.5 cm) (sheet)
1989-69-68

74
Trade Card for
**C. Owen, Chemist, Druggist & Tea
Dealer**
English, late nineteenth century
Engraving
2¹/₂ x 3⁵/₈″ (6.4 x 9.2 cm)
1989-69-51

75
Trade Card for
G. Owen Man-midwife
English, late nineteenth century
Engraving
2³/₄ x 4¹/₄″ (6.9 x 10.8 cm)
1989-69-33

Trade cards of British merchants and
other professionals often included
emblems of their activities. Arnold's
card (no. 72) is a detailed view of
the facade of his pharmacy in Norwich, and the illustration on the card
for S. Moss (no. 73) of Cheltenham
shows a scale and chemical apparatus used in the manufacture of
several of his products. On his card
C. Owen (no. 74), chemist, druggist,
and tea dealer of Abingdon, also
includes appropriate symbolism: a
retort and a Chinese figure resting
before a temple. The drawing on
man-midwife G. Owen's card (no.
75) is appropriately of a mother
holding her child and a father whose
arrow has slain a threatening snake.

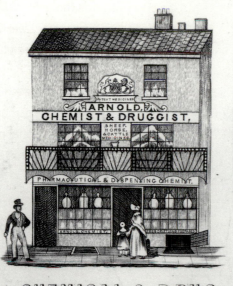

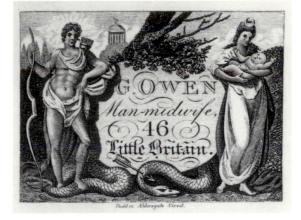

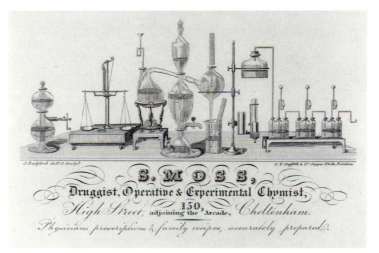

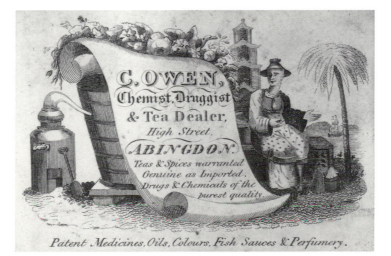

76
Trade Card for
**Etablissement Hydrosudopathique
du Docteur de Cock**
Belgian, Ghent, 1840–65
Color lithograph on coated paper
4¹⁵/₁₆ x 6⁷/₈" (12.5 x 17.5 cm)
(sheet)
1988-102-107

This "porcelain" card (see no. 77)
shows the principal buildings of the
"hydrosudopathique" spa operated
by Dr. de Cock at Grammont, a small
village in Belgium between Brussels
and Courtrai. Certainly the presence
of hydrogen sulfide in the water gave
it an unpleasant odor and taste;
entrepreneurs such as Dr. de Cock
claimed that such waters were beneficial in the treatment of various
ailments, primarily the rheumatic.
In addition to the possible good
imparted by taking the waters, considerable added benefit probably
derived from the rest one obtained in
such an establishment.

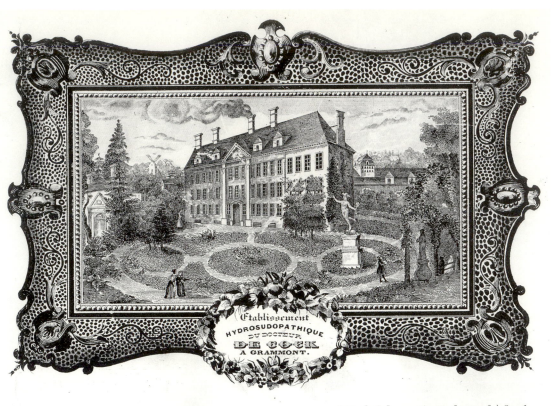

77
Trade Card for
C. B. Geeraert, Pharmacien
Belgian, Bruges, c. 1875
Color lithograph on coated paper
4½ x 6¹¹/₁₆" (11.4 x 17 cm)
1988-102-46

The trade card of the Belgian pharmacist C. B. Geeraert is an example
of a "porcelain" card, one printed on
paper made by a process incorporat-
ing white lead. This technique gave
the card a special gloss that resem-
bled the transparent glaze of undec-
orated porcelain, and enabled the
lithographs to appear as engravings.
Belgium was the center of the "porcelain" card industry. In this example, a large mortar and pestle,
medicinal plants, and a distillation
apparatus, symbols of the pharmacist's profession, have been appropriately incorporated into the
design.

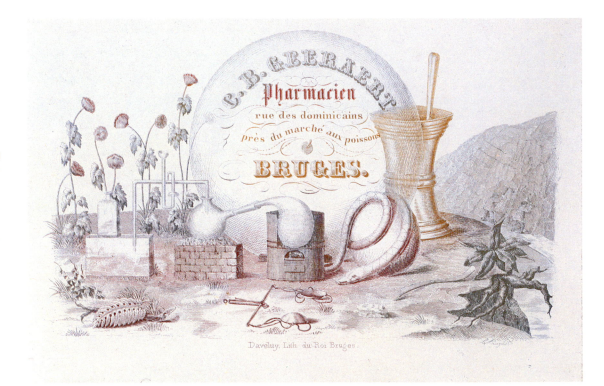

78
Trade Card for
D. Goethals, Pharmacien
Belgian, Ghent, c. 1875
Lithograph on coated paper
4⁷/₁₆ x 6¹/₈" (11.3 x 15.6 cm)
(sheet)
1988-102-129

The pharmacist D. Goethals prepared this card to announce the
relocation of his pharmacy in Ghent.
Under a stag holding a mortar and
pestle are rows of shelves filled with
apothecary jars, with a distillation
scene added to the pharmaceutical
images at the bottom. Like many
nineteenth-century broadsides, each
line in the announcement is printed
in a different type face.

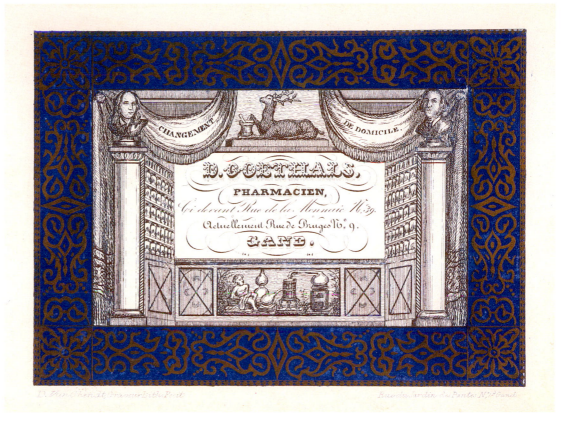

79
Trade Card for
**Pharmacie & Droguerie de
A. G. Lancksweert**
Belgian, Ghent, c. 1875
Lithograph on coated paper
4¹/₂ x 6³/₁₆" (11.4 x 15.7 cm)
(sheet)
1988-102-108

The alembic and other parts of a
distillation apparatus are the only
symbols on this "porcelain" card
that directly relate to the business of
A. G. Lancksweert, the proprietor of
a pharmacy in Ghent. Although
several of the other emblems,
including the bust (which may be
Hippocrates), the snake, and the
stag, might also have medical rele-
vance, their iconography is so general that the large box in the center
of the card could have contained
imprints for other, nonmedical
businesses.

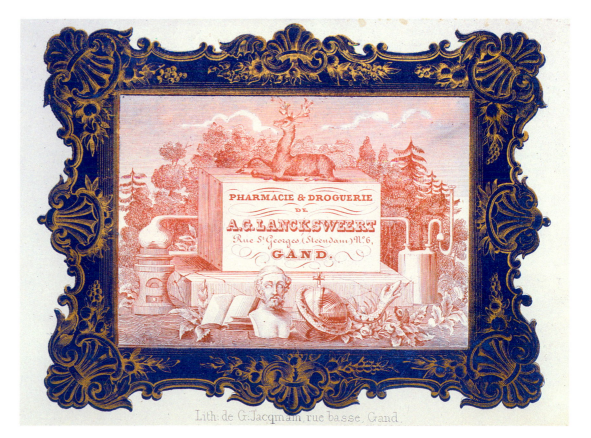

80

Trade Card for
Bright's Kidney Beans
American, late nineteenth century
Color lithograph with relief printing
on coated paper
6⅛ x 4⅜" (15.5 x 11.1 cm)
1989-8-7

When it is folded, the card advertising Bright's Kidney Beans looks like a clam shell, and like the mollusk, only reveals its merit when opened. The company that made the pills declared them to be the "Best Kidney, Liver and Backache Cure In the World," at a time when little was known about how to treat such problems. The use of the name "Bright's" was probably an attempt to suggest the product's utility in the treatment of Bright's disease, a serious condition affecting the kidneys.

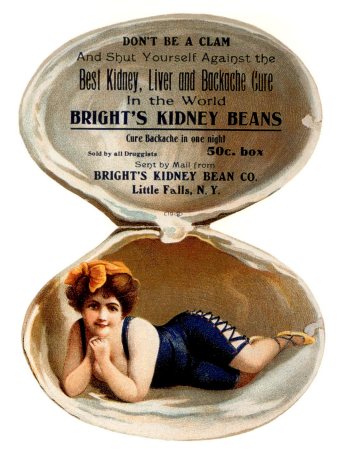

81

Trade Card for
Las Grajeas Dubourg and
El Hemoneurol Cognet
French, late nineteenth century
Color lithograph with relief printing
on coated paper
2¹³⁄₁₆ x 4⅛" (7.2 x 10.5 cm)
1989-8-65

Stock card series were published with hundreds of subjects, some of which could be considered appropriate for proprietary medicines and others that might seem to be less than fitting. The set illustrating the martyrdom of saints, represented here by the example with Saint Dionysus, is clearly in the second category, yet the Cognet company used the cards to promote two of their products, Dubourg pills for constipation and Hemoneurol for improved strength and vigor.

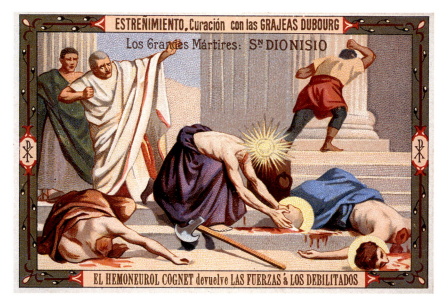

82
Trade Cards for
Cognet Medicines
French, late nineteenth century
Color lithographs
each 4¹/₂ x 2⁷/₈″ (11.4 x 7.3 cm)
1989-8-25–27, 29

The Cognet firm was based in Paris and its main market was France, but its products were distributed to other European countries as well. This set of trade cards, for example, carried Spanish text within Art Nouveau illustrations of women representing flowers. Among the products advertised were Cognet capsules for coughs (the rose and chrysanthemum cards), Dubourg pills for constipation (the iris card), and iron pills for anemia (the wisteria card).

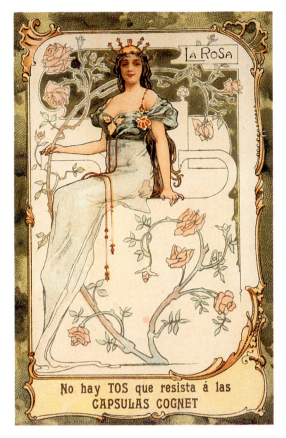

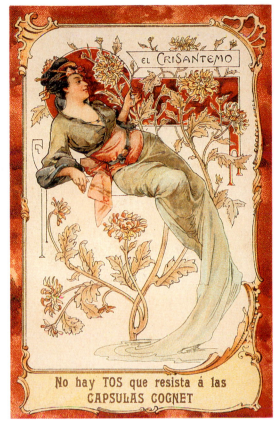

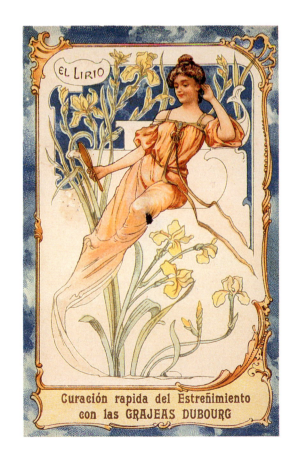

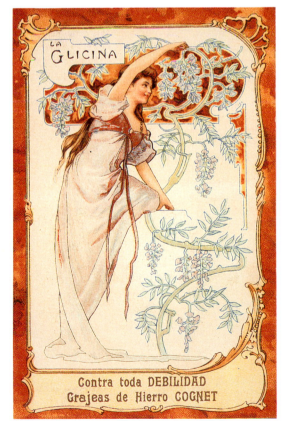

83
Trade Card for
English Female Bitters
American, Louisville, Kentucky, late
nineteenth century
Color relief print
5¼ x 3⅛" (13.3 x 7.9 cm)
1989-8-67

The young woman is being served a
dose of English Female Bitters by
her maid in a depiction of the relationship between different social
classes that was unusual in the
egalitarian world of nineteenth-
century America. The bitters were
promoted for "the cure of all female
complaints," a blanket term that
included premenstrual tension,
leukorrhea, prolapsed uterus, ovar-
ian disorders, and vaginal bleeding.
Because of the reluctance of women
to consult with physicians, many
products were marketed as promised
cures for such problems. Few, however, could match the claims of this
product, which advertised that it
"assists nature in toning and building up the feeble and flagging ener-
gies, . . . imparts vitality, adds
lustre to the eye, brilliancy to the
intellect, gladness to the heart and
restores women to strength, health
and happiness."

84
Trade Cards for
Berlingots-Eysséric
French, late nineteenth century
Color lithographs with relief printing
each 4¹/₁₆ x 2⁹/₁₆" (10.3 x 6.5 cm)
1989-8-1, 3

Berlingots, the French word for
small sweets made with caramel,
are a specialty of Carpentras in
the Vaucluse region of France. In
addition to being pleasant-tasting
lozenges, they also have been
recommended for digestive disorders and seasickness. The Eysséric
company marketed one of the leading brands of *berlingots* and was
also a major user of trade cards as
an advertising medium. Among the
series they issued were cards with
information on the planets, such as
these examples on Jupiter and
Mercury. The image of the latter is
based on Giovanni da Bologna's
well-known sculpture (Museo
Nazionale del Bargello, Florence).

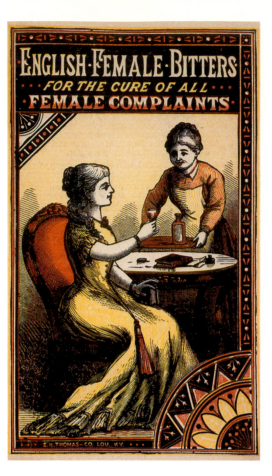

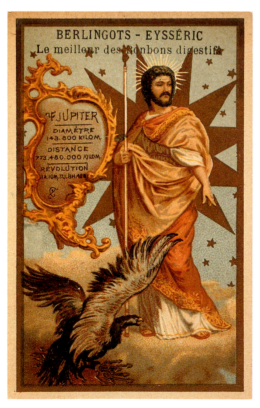

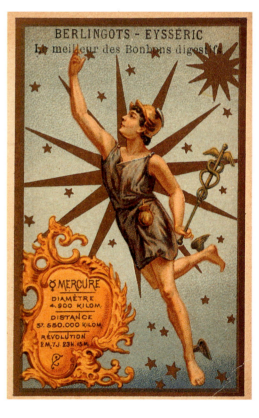

85
Trade Cards for
Faricum Medicines
American, New York, late nineteenth
century
Color lithographs
each 3 x 4⁷/₈″ (7.6 x 12.3 cm)
1989-8-69—71

The images on trade cards for the
three Faricum specialties illustrate
one of the staples of pharmaceutical
advertising, and one that has been
adopted so successfully by television: the before-and-after picture.
By applying Faricum Almandine, a
woman sees her freckles quickly
disappear; by taking Faricum Cough
Drops, an actress is able to go on
stage; and by using Faricum for the
cure of diphtheria, sore throat,
croup, and catarrh, an entire city has
been made well. In the latter, the
artist's skill at depicting a multitude
of people in the small space of the
card is especially evident.

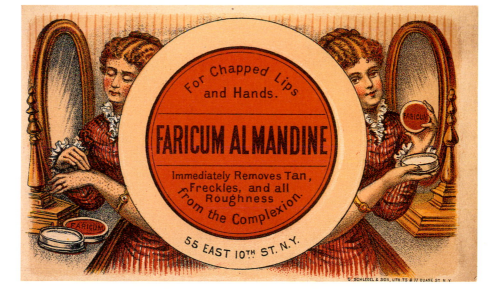

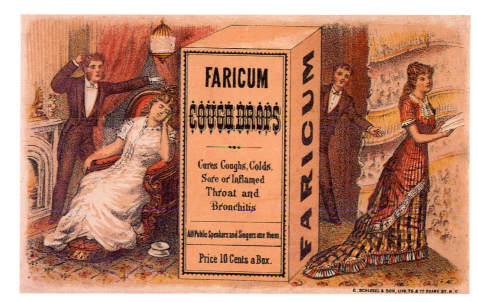

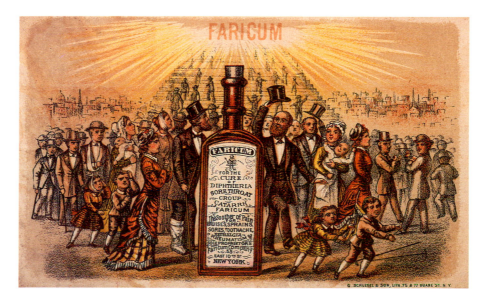

86
Trade Cards for
Fernet-Branca
Italian, Milan, late nineteenth
century
Color lithographs
each approximately 5¼ x 3½"
(13.3 x 8.9 cm)
1989-8-72—74

A disproportionately large bottle of
Fernet-Branca is prominently displayed on each of these three cards,
one held by an eagle on a globe, a
second supporting a languid woman,
and a third on a pedestal behind an
American and a French woman who
toast one another. Still popular,
Fernet-Branca is used to treat indigestion, and its manufacturer,
Fratelli Branca of Milan, also has
recommended it on occasion for
treating intermittent fevers and for
expelling worms.

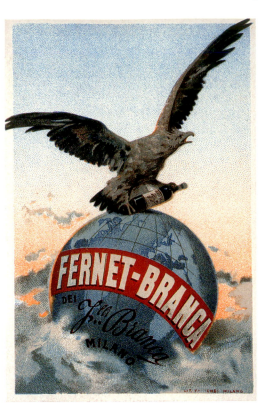

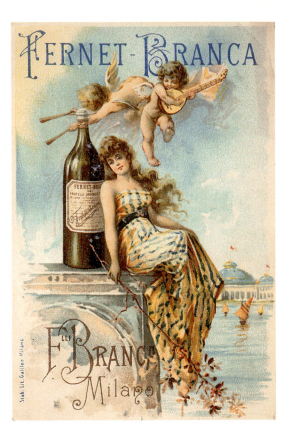

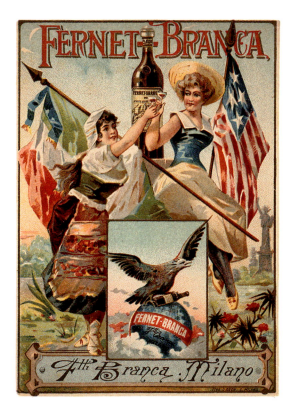

87

Trade Card for
**Hall's Vegetable Sicilian Hair
Renewer**
American, New York, late nineteenth
century
Color lithograph on coated paper
3⁹⁄₁₆ x 8¹⁄₁₆" (9.1 x 20.5 cm)
1989-8-77

"Five attractive faces" from Japan,
Holland, "dear America," Persia,
and Spain, "differing widely in their
graces," illustrate the virtues of
Hall's Vegetable Sicilian Hair
Renewer, a product that promised to
thicken hair, restore gray hair to its
original color, cure dandruff, and
prevent baldness. Reuben P. Hall,
its manufacturer, had obtained
the formula, as he testified, from
a destitute sailor whom he had
befriended; the product contained
sulfur and lead acetate as hair
restoratives in addition to glycerin,
boroglycerin, capsicum, rosemary,
bay rum, and tea in a solution of 15
percent alcohol.

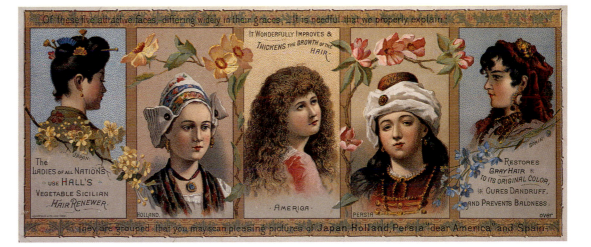

88

Trade Card for
**Hibbard's Rheumatic Syrup and
Plaster**
American, after 1885
Color lithograph
3¹⁄₄ x 5¹⁄₂" (8.2 x 14 cm)
1989-8-79

Maud S. was one of trotting's immor-
tals; her fastest time for the mile was
2:08³⁄₄ minutes, set at a track in
Cleveland in 1885. Here her speed
is used to advertise the rapidity with
which Hibbard's Rheumatic Syrup
would go to work as the "most effective remedy for Rheumatism, General Debility, Affections of the heart,
and all diseases arising from Impure
Blood." The jockey holds aloft both a
Hibbard's Rheumatic Plaster and a
bottle of the syrup, which immod-
estly claimed to be "a panacea for all
blood diseases," and had been
formulated from roots and herbs by
Chloe Hibbard, a nurse and "botani-
cal physician" practicing in Butler,
New York.

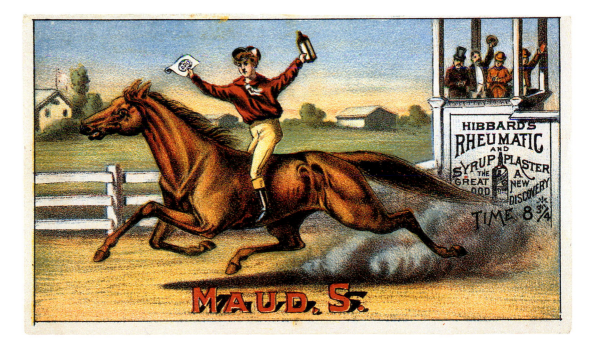

89
Trade Cards for
Hop Pills
American, New London, Connecticut,
late nineteenth century
Lithographs with relief printing
each 4½ x 2⅝" (11.4 x 6.6 cm)
1989-8-80—85

Portraits of the well known contemporary stage performers Bessie Clayton, Effie Ellsler, Mary Garden, Maude Branscombe, Venie Clancey, and Emma Thursby appear on this set of black-and-white stock cards used in this case to advertise Hop Pills. While hops, the dried ripe cones of the female flowers of the Humulus plant, still find use in brewing, their medicinal attributes are no longer believed to be particularly strong, and cannot live up to the promise, printed on the reverse of the cards, that "they are a wonderful Tonic, Narcotic and Diuretic, and are highly useful in the cure of all Liver, Nerve and Kidney Troubles, Biliousness, Weak Nerves, Dyspepsia, Neuralgia," and numerous other ailments.

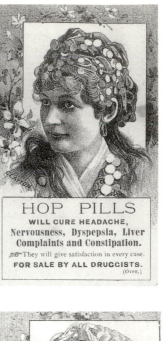
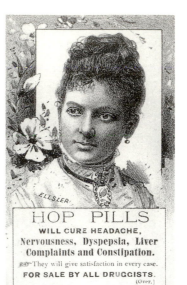
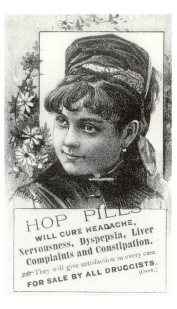
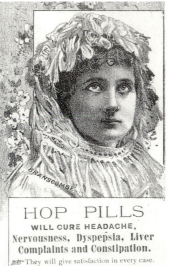
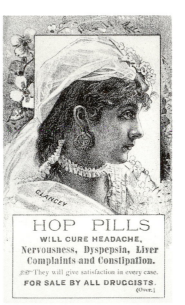
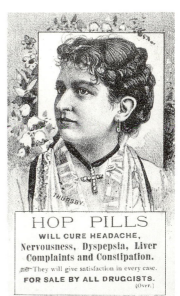

90
Trade Cards for
Jackson's Best
American, Five Points, New York,
late nineteenth century
Color lithographs
each 5⅛ x 3⁷⁄₁₆" (13 x 8.7 cm)
1989-8-88—94

A series of cartoons, in a sequential
form similar to that of contemporary
comic strips, tells of "How Adolphus
Slim-Jim Used Jackson's Best
[Chewing Tobacco] and Was Happy."
In two of the illustrations a physician
takes the patient's pulse, diagnoses
the young man's lovesickness, and
prescribes Jackson's tobacco, which
leads to a happy ending to the story.
Originally published as part of a
booklet, each card includes a sizable
advertisement for Jackson's Best to
reinforce its message and to insure
continued publicity in case the
pages were separated.

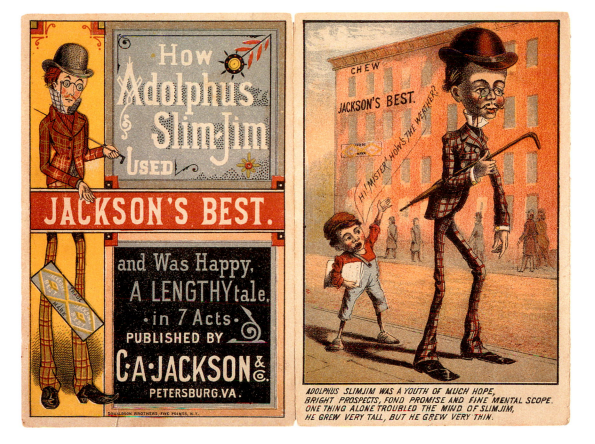

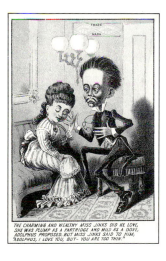

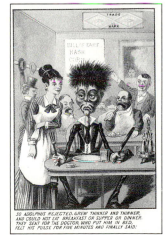

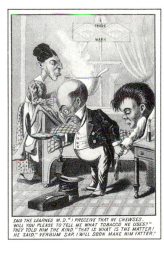

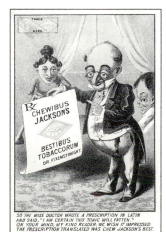

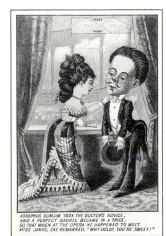

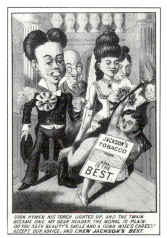

91
Trade Card for
Pildoras Sanativas de Jayne
Possibly Spanish, late nineteenth
century
Color lithograph on coated paper
5½ x 4⅜" (14 x 11.1 cm)
1989-8-135

An angel, evocative of Gabriel and his horn, advertises Jayne's Sanative Pills, a product that acted as a mild laxative in small doses of one to three pills, and as a potent cathartic in larger amounts. During the 1860s, long before federal legislation curtailed the excesses of medical advertisements, these pills were recommended for liver complaints, gout, jaundice, and nineteen additional conditions. Their manufacturer, Dr. David Jayne, began to market medicines in Philadelphia in 1830, and his first advertisements appeared in 1849. These cards were printed in Spanish for distribution in Latin America, a major export region for the company.

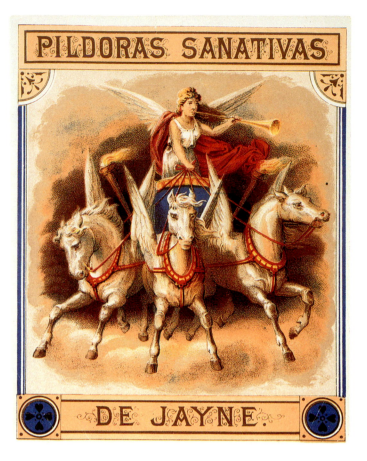

92
Trade Card for
Dr. Kilmer's Ocean-Weed Heart Remedy
American, New York, late nineteenth
century
Color lithograph
3¹/₁₆ x 5³/₁₆" (7.8 x 13.2 cm)
1989-8-50

A series of theatrically displayed pastoral views were used to promote products marketed by Dr. Kilmer & Co. of Binghamton, New York. A maritime setting has been chosen for the Ocean-Weed Heart Remedy, which was recommended if the "heart thumps after sudden effort, skips beats or flutters," as well as for edema, vertigo, neuralgia, and other ailments.

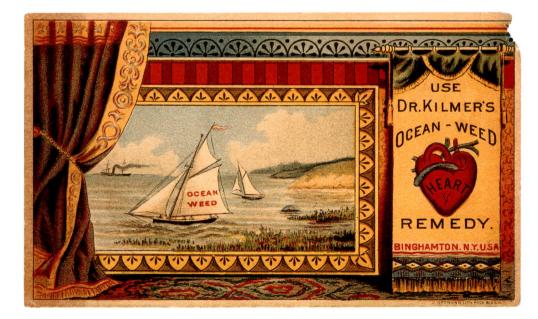

93
Trade Cards for
Liebig Products
Belgian, Antwerp, late nineteenth
century
Color lithographs on coated paper
each 4½ x 2¹³⁄₁₆″ (11.4 x 7.2 cm)
1990-104-1—6

The chief product of the Liebig
company was a concentrated meat
extract that was marketed throughout Europe and the Americas. Purchasers of the extract received
tokens that could be exchanged for
a series of cards such as this set on
the applied arts; each card also
shows an illustration of the product's
package. Liebig encouraged people
to collect the cards by also providing
albums for the sets. In some in-
stances information on the images
appeared on the reverse of the card,
but in the majority of cases, as in
these examples, recipes incorporat-
ing one of the Liebig products were
given. This set, one of approximately
two thousand series of chromolithographed trade cards on hundred of
subjects that the company issued
between 1872 and 1974, was
published in Antwerp.

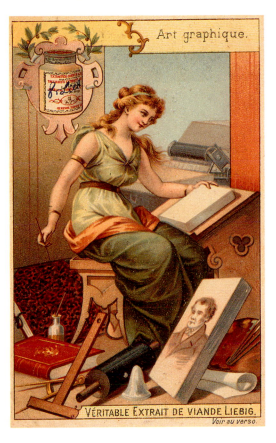

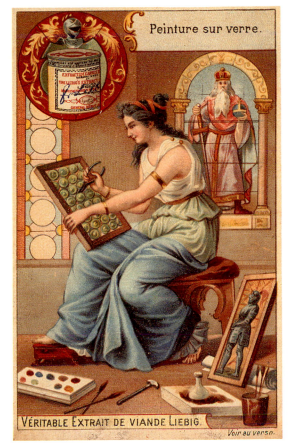

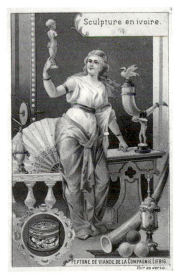

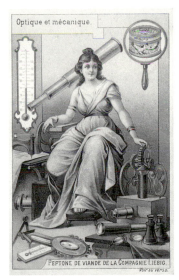

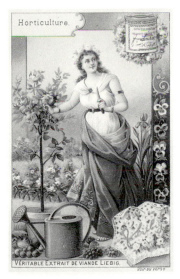

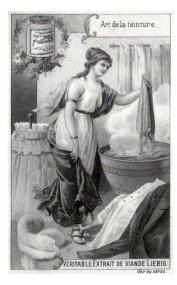

94

Trade Card for
Firma C. Lück
German, 1890–1900
Color lithograph on coated paper
5⅞ x 4″ (14.9 x 10.2 cm)
1989-8-37

Portraits of six prominent members of the German Reichstag between 1893 and 1898 surround an imperial eagle on a card that promotes products of the C. Lück company of Colberg (now Kołobrzeg, Poland). The eminent legislators are Hans von Kanitz-Podangen, Berthold von Ploetz-Döllingen, Karl von Stumm, Klemens von Heeremann, Ernst Lieber, and Franz Hitze; their political party affiliations are also noted. On the reverse of the card are advertisements for three products distributed by the company, the principal one being a topical antirheumatic containing camphor, henbane, ether, and pine needle oil.

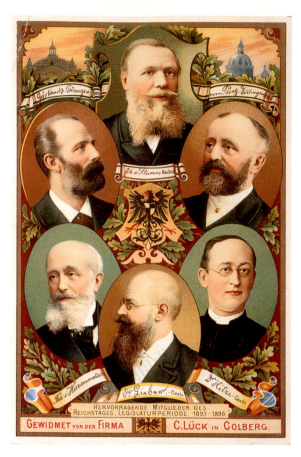

95

Trade Cards for
Lutted's Cough Drops
American, Buffalo, late nineteenth century
Color lithographs
each 5¼ x 3½″ (13.3 x 8.9 cm)
1989-8-104, 105

Scenes of winter sports, walking on snowshoes and tobogganing, are put to use to advertise Lutted's Cough Drops. The illustrations are appropriate for a product used frequently in winter months, but there is no additional text to associate them with this medication. Although most nineteenth-century trade cards bear extravagant discussions of the benefits of the product advertised, in this case the name alone was deemed to be sufficient.

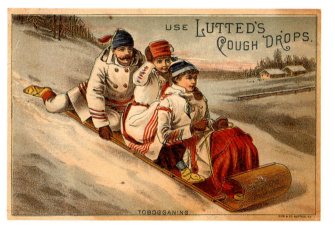

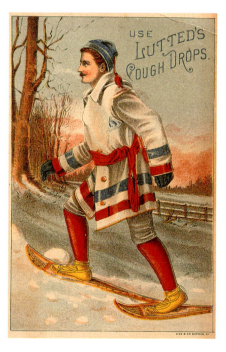

96
Bookmarks for
Mennen's Powders
American, early twentieth century
Color lithographs on coated paper
each approximately 6 x 2"
(15.5 x 5 cm)
1989-8-108—110

In their promotional campaigns, the
Mennen Chemical Company used an
assortment of bookmarks such as
the three shown to proclaim the
virtues of their medicated powders.
The Borated Talcum Toilet Powder
was "recommended by the leading
physicians and nurses to relieve
Prickly Heat, Nettle Rash, Sunburn,
Chafing and all skin affections," and
the Sen-Yang Powder was formulated without starch, rice, or other
irritants. Even the Flesh Tint Talcum, illustrated with a woman
admiring herself in a mirror, had all
the medicinal and antiseptic quali-
ties of the borated varieties.

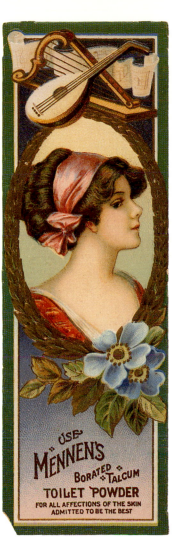

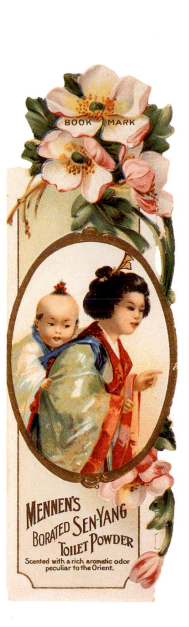

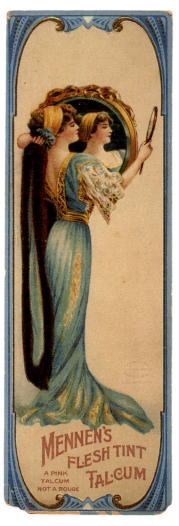

97
Trade Card for
Dr. Morse's Indian Root Pills and
Comstock's Dead Shot Worm Pellets
American, late nineteenth century
Color lithograph
4⅝ x 3″ (11.8 x 7.6 cm)
1989-8-56

The Indian warrior on his rearing horse, ready to slay a menacing bear, was a symbol for Dr. Morse's Indian Root Pills, one of many proprietary medicines that claimed to be based on formulas obtained from Native Americans. Groups such as the Indians were surrounded by an aura of exotic mystery in the popular imagination and hence were continuously used to promote medicines, for products said to have originated with them were thought to have special healing power. The composition of Dr. Morse's pills varied over time, but usually contained a mixture of organic laxatives such as aloes, mandrake, gamboge, jalap, podophyllin, and cayenne pepper. The Indian Root Pills were the major product of the W. H. Comstock Company, which has here added an advertisement for its Dead Shot Worm Pellets, which had no connection with Indians, below the illustration.

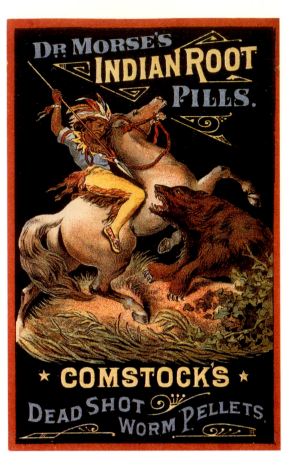

98
Trade Cards for
Nichols' Bark and Iron
American, c. 1884
Color lithographs on coated paper
each 5½ x 3½″ (14 x 8.9 cm)
1989-8-116, 117

Along with attractive women and domestic scenes, children were among the most popular images used in nineteenth-century American advertising trade cards. In this example, well-dressed children advertise a product that contained iron and quinine, and was recommended for several conditions, including loss of appetite, indigestion, malaria, and even hypochondria. Nichols' Bark and Iron claimed to be "especially adapted for Clergymen, Counsellors, Journalists, and persons of sedentary habits." Certainly the iron the tonic contained could be expected to be beneficial in cases of anemia and the quinine in treating malaria, but the product could not have been as useful for other conditions for which it was recommended.

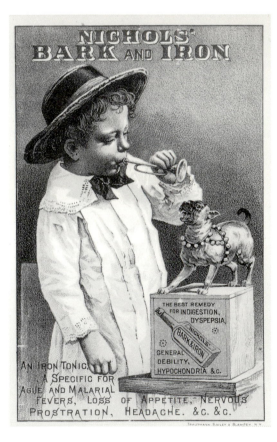

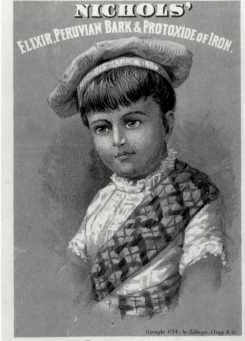

99
Trade Cards for
Pharmacie Normale
French, Paris, late nineteenth
century
Color lithographs
each 4³⁄₈ x 3″ (11.1 x 7.6 cm)
1989-8-130, 131

Trade cards tracing the evolution of
military uniforms carried advertising
for the Pharmacie Normale, a successful business in Paris that used
such cards as its primary means of
publicity. The reverse of the cards
lists cosmetics and requisites for
dental hygiene as well as other
specialties of the pharmacy, such
as the Glycérine Anglaise of Dr.
Schmith.

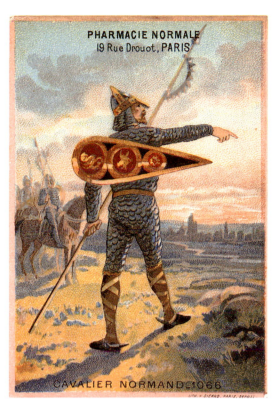

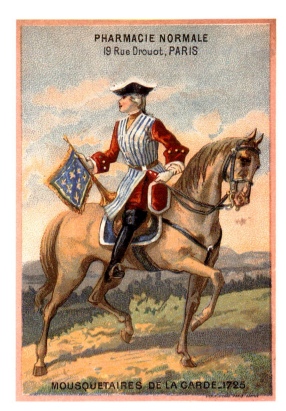

100
Trade Card for
Pike's Toothache Drops
American, late nineteenth century
Color lithograph
5 x 3″ (12.7 x 7.6 cm)
1989-8-134

The drawing of a dentist applying
Pike's Toothache Drops to his patient
confirms professional acceptance
of the product, which, according to
the text on the reverse of the card,
promises to "annihilate in one
minute the most violent and protracted toothache," and to "cure
nervous toothache when rubbed
behind the sufferer's ears." The
drops were made of natural ingredients, the chief of which was probably morphine or another opium
derivative.

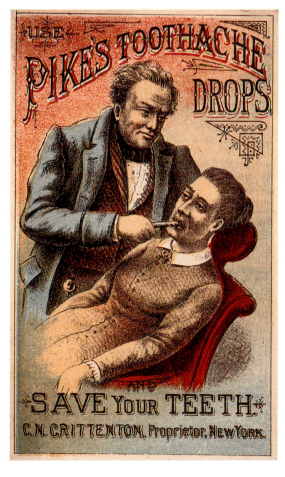

101
Trade Card for
Sapanule
American, Providence, Rhode
Island, after 1878
Color lithograph
2¹/₂ x 4¹/₁₆" (6.4 x 10.3 cm)
1989-8-145

In a design quite advanced for its
period, Oriental figures were used
on this trade card advertising
Sapanule, a glycerin-based lotion.
Not only was this product promoted
as a cure for neuralgia, diphtheria,
and rheumatism, but it also was said
to be useful in treating erysipelas,
eczema, and pneumonia. Since
nineteenth-century therapeutics
were generally more concerned with
restoring proper balance than with
using specific drugs to treat specific
illnesses, it was not unusual for a
product to claim to be effective
against a variety of conditions.

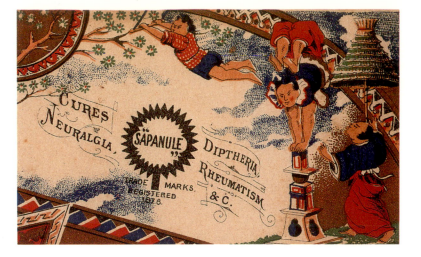

102
Trade Card for
Dr. Scott's Bilious & Liver Pills
English, after 1901
Color lithograph on coated paper
6⁷/₈ x 4³/₈" (17.5 x 11.1 cm)
1989-8-61

A clown balances a package of Dr.
Scott's Bilious & Liver Pills on his
toe, controlling it in such a way that
the label on the box can be easily
read. Scott's Pills were unequaled as
a general family aperient medicine,
as the advertisement on the reverse
of the card noted, and were claimed
to "give a healthy tone and vigour to
the different secretions, causing the
necessary organs of the Stomach
and Liver to resume their activity,
thus restoring the appetite."

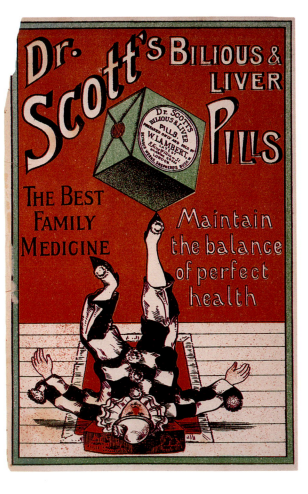

103

Trade Cards for
Star Cough Drops
American, late nineteenth century
Color lithographs with relief printing
on coated paper
each 4¼ x 2½" (10.8 x 6.4 cm)
1989-8-148, 149

The singer and the bassist are part of
a series of six cards with images of
performers quoting lines from Gil-
bert and Sullivan's *Patience*, which
were published shortly after the
comic opera was first performed in
1881. *Patience* lampooned the
popularity of Oscar Wilde and similarly caricatured the Aesthetic
Movement that he personified. On
these cards, the makers of Star
Cough Drops turned this aspect of
the musical to their advantage by
boasting that "All 'Aesthetic' People" use their product. The cards in
the *Patience* series were known as
stock cards, for they were kept in a
printer's stock and imprinted with
advertisements for all types of
commercial products, not only
medicines.

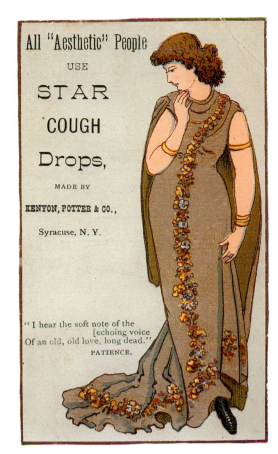

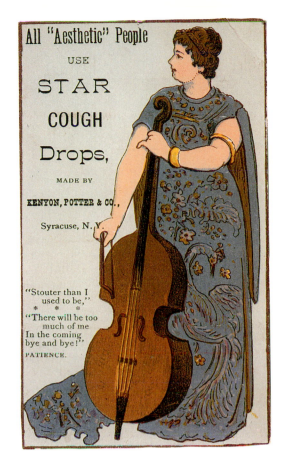

104

Trade Cards for
Tapioca de l'Etoile
French, Paris, after 1889
Color lithographs on coated paper
each 4³⁄₁₆ x 2¹¹⁄₁₆" (10.6 x 6.8 cm)
1988-102-15, 22

The late nineteenth-century equiva-
lent of modern baseball cards were
chromolithographed cards of important events and famous people,
including notable scientists and
medical practitioners; the reverse
of such cards contained information
on the contributions made by these
individuals. Examples include these
cards of Andreas Vesalius, the
anatomist who made extensive use
of dissection in delineating the
structure and function of the human
body; and Philippe Pinel, the French
physician who pioneered in the
humane treatment of the insane.

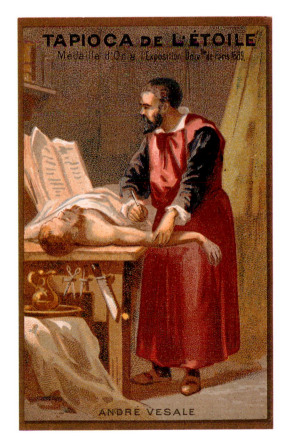

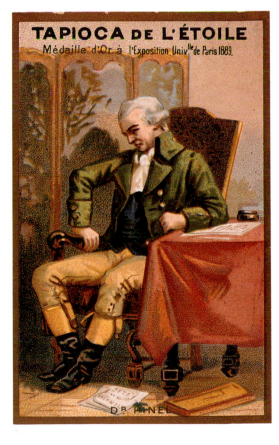

105

Trade Cards for
Ten Eyck and Browne, Druggists
American, late nineteenth century
Color lithographs on coated paper
each 4¾ x 4¹/₁₆" (12.1 x 10.3 cm)
1989-8-153, 155

Stock cards were available in an
almost endless range of shapes and
sizes. The firm of Craig and Elliot
printed these fan-shaped trade cards
illustrated with children's faces. The
designer did not leave sufficient
blank space for text, however, and
thus the names of Ten Eyck and
Browne, the proprietors of the City
Drug Store in Cohoes, New York, are
difficult to decipher amidst the
decoration on the fans.

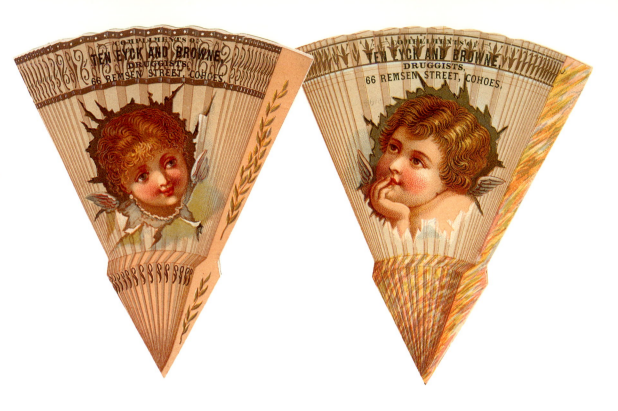

106

Trade Cards for
Warner's Safe Yeast
American, Rochester, New York,
late nineteenth century
Color lithographs on coated paper
each 5⁷/₁₆ x 3¹⁵/₁₆" (13.8 x 10 cm)
1989-8-163, 165

Early in his career, Herbert Har-
rington Warner was a distributor
of safes for a firm that eventually
became the Mosler Safe Company.
When he later began to manufacture
a line of proprietary remedies, he
appropriated the word "safe" for
many of his products, including
Warner's Safe Yeast, to convey a
guarantee of security. He frequently
illustrated an iron safe on the labels,
as seen here, and similar safes were
molded in relief on the blown-glass
bottles of other products. Warner's
large plant and office building,
shown on one of these trade cards,
still stands in Rochester. The other
card suggests that the advertised
product provides "safe" passage
between the perilous straits of
"Indigestion" and "Bad Health,"
which are represented as rock forma-
tions shaped as grotesque heads.

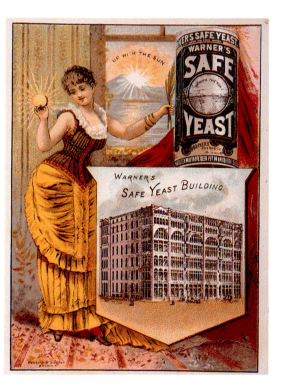

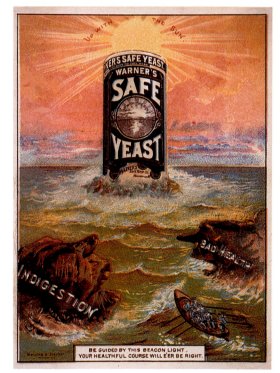

107
Advertisement for
Carpenter's Chemical Warehouse
Frontispiece from George
Washington Carpenter, *Essays on Some of the Most Important Articles of the Materia Medica*, 2nd ed., rev. and enl. (Philadelphia, 1834)
Engraving
8¼ x 5¼" (21 x 13.3 cm)
1989-69-26

The advertisement showing the facade of Carpenter's Chemical Warehouse at Eighth and Market streets in Philadelphia appeared as the frontispiece to the second edition of a collection of essays by George Washington Carpenter, a druggist who also sold chemical and scientific apparatus. Not only are the names of many popular products listed on this print, but, rather surprisingly in an age of secret remedies, the contents of some of them are also revealed. The head of Aesculapius over the bow window represents a continuation of the seventeenth- and eighteenth-century British custom of using the busts of such famous figures from the history of medicine on apothecary shops, a useful device when homes and stores were not yet given street numbers and illiteracy was widespread.

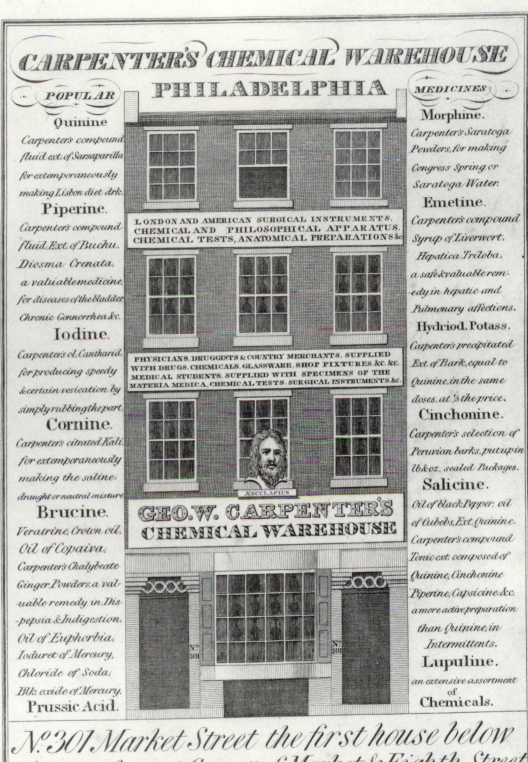

108
Advertisement for
Shiseido Pharmacy
Chikanobu Toyohara (Yoshu)
(Japanese, 1838—1912)
1878
Color woodcut
14½ x 9¾" (36.8 x 24.8 cm)
(sheet, cropped within margin)
1988-102-35

These three physicians are confer-
ring at the Shiseido pharmacy in
Tokyo, discussing the merits of the
company's products. Two are from
the army, Dr. Yoshi Hayashi, the
third chief military physician (left),
and Dr. Jun Matsumoto, the second
chief military physician (right). In
the center is Dr. Naonaka Sato, the
head of the pharmacy. The large
horizontal panel on the wall states
that people become ill when they are
not examined by good physicians,
that treatment is often too expen-
sive, and that Shiseido has developed good products, one of which
was given to a sick person by the
Meiji emperor while on an inspection
tour. Vertical banners advertise
various products of the pharmacy.

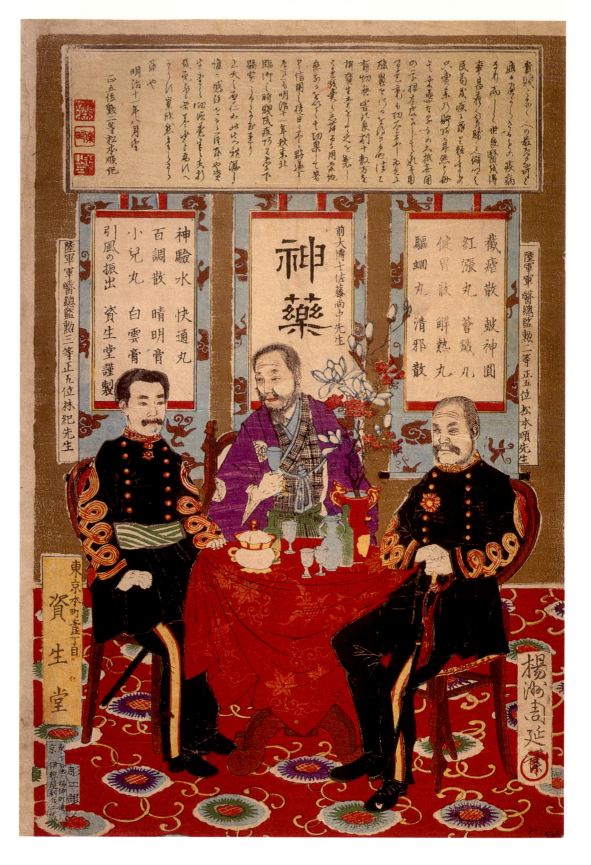

109
Advertisement for
Rakuzendo Pharmacy
Eitaku (Japanese, 1843–1890)
1880–90
Color woodcut
13¹¹⁄₁₆ x 9³⁄₈" (34.8 x 23.8 cm)
(sheet)
1988-102-36

A woman and child read advertisements for medicines on two large scrolls. The scroll on the left discusses the indications and merits of three products sold by the Rakuzendo pharmacy in Tokyo: On-Tsu-Gan, pills for constipation that were pleasant in their action; Chin-Ryu-In, a potion that was useful in various problems of the gastrointestinal tract; and Ho-Yo-Gan, pills for improving strength and well-being in several conditions, such as following childbirth. The other scroll advertises Sei-Ki-Sui, an ophthalmic product developed by an American physician.

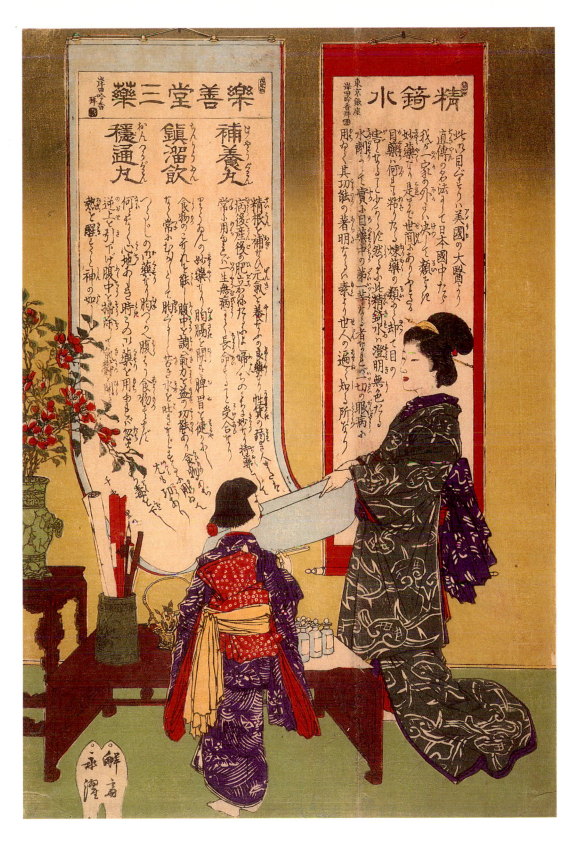

110
Popular Prints
**Las Desgracias de Pedrín
(The Misfortunes of Pedrín)**
Spanish, c. 1860
Relief prints
each sheet approximately 16½ x
11¼″ (41.9 x 28.6 cm)
1988-102-37, 38

Twenty-four scenes in the unhappy life of Pedrín illustrate his sufferings from such misfortunes as seasickness, toothache, nosebleed, and chilblains. The popular images in these two prints are derived from *Le Médecin à la maison*, a large colored engraving from the *Encyclopédie Bouasse-Lebel* ([Paris, c. 1860], no. 61) giving directions for simple treatments for the illnesses and accidents of daily life. Each subject in the earlier French print is repeated here in the Spanish versions, but with the order changed and with crudely drawn images replacing the more elegant originals. The text, however, rather than being a home health guide, has been changed into a simple tale of an ill-starred victim. Thus a text explaining the causes and treatments of the ailment of a gouty gentleman is sharply altered to a brief verse stating that Pedrín had overeaten; similarly a list of the first-aid measures that accompanies an image of an asphyxiated patient is changed to a complaint that Pedrín has become indolent.

(Núm. 115.)

LAS DESGRACIAS DE PEDRIN.—SEGUNDA PARTE

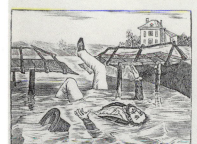

13 Al atravesar un puente
para meterse en el puerto
se cayó del puente abajo
y se quedó medio muerto.

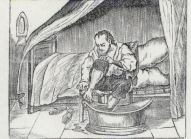

14 Todo lleno de chichones,
para curarse su mal,
el infeliz D. Pedrín,
se metió en el hospital.

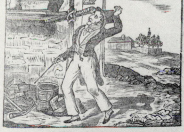

15 Le mandaron pasear,
estando convaleciente,
y la punta de un andamio
hizo pedazos su frente.

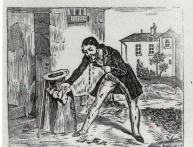

16 Por reprender á los chicos
que le echaban agua á chorros,
á tronchazos y pedradas
le deshicieron los morros.

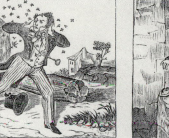

17 Era goloso Pedrín
y por hartarse de miel
las abejas le picaron
y se cebaron en él.

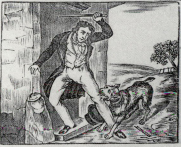

18 El guardian de las colmenas
le desgarró el pantalón
y Pedrin hizo pedazos
en su cabeza el bastón.

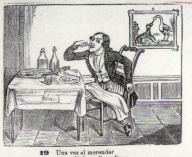

19 Una vez al merendar
se comió dos mil sardinas
y tuvo que estar tres meses
sacándose las espinas.

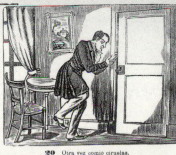

20 Otra vez comió ciruelas,
creyó llegado su fin
pues toda la noche anduvo
desde la cama al bacín.

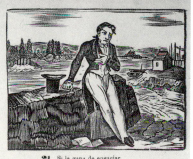

21 Si la gana de ensuciar
de pronto le acometía
se bajaba el pantalón
y en el sombrero lo hacia.

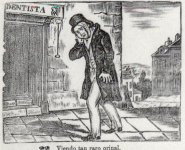

22 Viendo tan raro orinal,
los revoltosos chiquillos
á pedradas le dejaron
sin dientes y sin colmillos.

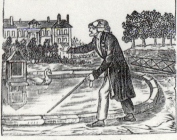

23 Tantos sustos y desgracias,
tanta falta de sosiego,
concluyeron por dejarle
desdichado, pobre y ciego.

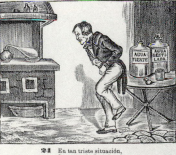

24 En tan triste situación,
desesperado Pedrín,
un veneno se tomó
y puso á su vida fin.

MADRID.—Despacho: Hernando, Arenal, 11.

111
Popular Print
Va-t-en voir s'ils viennent, Jean, ou Les Raretés (Go See If They Are Coming, Jean, or The Rarities)
French, Epinal, c. 1880
Hand-colored relief print
11¹/₁₆ x 15⁷/₁₆" (28.1 x 39.2 cm)
1988-102-27

The apothecary, his clyster at the ready, dutifully awaits the physician's signal to administer its contents when the examination is over. The hand-colored print is accompanied by verses to a song, *Go See If They Are Coming, Jean*, which satirizes an idealized society. For example, the doctor does not use long words, prescribes very little, and lets nature perform the cure. The print was published by the Pellerin workshop at Epinal, France, the largest supplier of *imagerie populaire*, or popular prints of artisanal manufacture on religious, historical, patriotic, educational, and humorous subjects that were distributed at low prices to the masses.

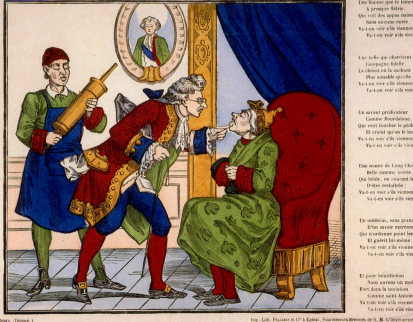

112
Envelope for
Lincoln's Laboratory
American, Salem, Massachusetts, c. 1864
Color relief print
3 x 5³/₈" (7.6 x 13.6 cm)
1988-102-6

During the Civil War, both the North and the South used envelopes as a medium for disseminating propaganda; in some cases half or more of the envelope was covered with an illustration, usually a caricature. In this multicolored example, Abraham Lincoln is at work in his laboratory, distilling off slavery from a mixture of Confederate states and cities to produce a "Pure Refined National Elixir of Liberty." Among the signs in the laboratory are several advertising medicines with the names of Lincoln's officers, including "[Robert Kingston?] Scott's Extirpation Powders Sure Cure for Rattlesnake Bite" and "[Benjamin] Butler's Mineral Pills." There is also a jar within which an effigy of Confederate President Jefferson Davis is hung.

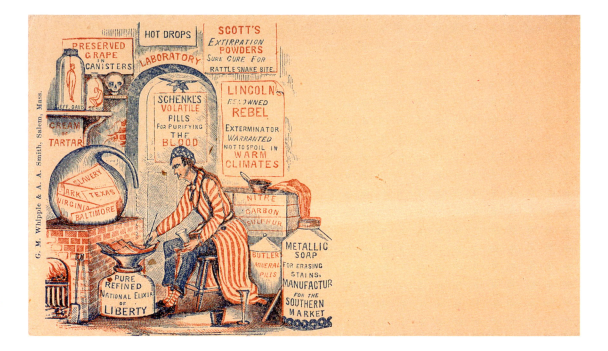

113
Stationery for
Armory Hospital, 1
American, 1861–65
Hand-colored lithograph
10³⁄₈ x 8¹⁄₄" (26.3 x 21 cm)
1988-102-1

114
Stationery for
**Columbia College & Carver Barracks
Hospitals 1**
American, 1861–65
Colored lithograph
10³⁄₈ x 8¹⁄₄" (26.3 x 21 cm)
1988-102-2

Lithographed images of hospitals
were used on stationery provided for
convalescing soldiers during the
Civil War. In the case of both the
Armory Hospital and the Columbia
College and Carver Barracks Hospitals in Washington, D.C., more than
one version was published, as the
number after the titles indicates.
The bird's-eye views show the unit-
and-pavilion system on which American military hospital architecture of
the 1860s was based; the advantage
of such a system was that a number
of small buildings could be con-
structed quickly to meet emergency
needs.

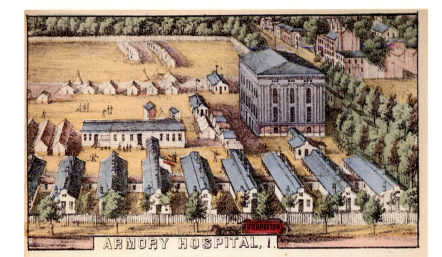

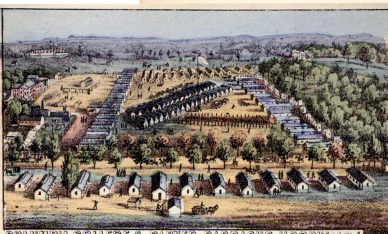

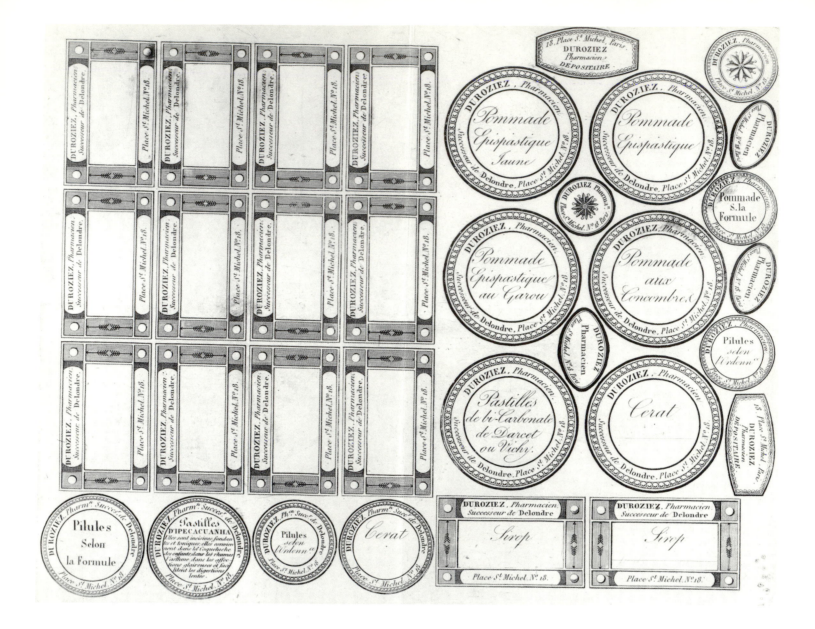

115
Labels for
Duroziez, Pharmacien
French, nineteenth century
Engraving
8¼ x 10³/₁₆″ (21 x 25.8 cm) (sheet)
1989-69-28

Until the twentieth century, most pharmacists' labels were printed on sheets, to be cut for use on individual prescriptions as needed (see also no. 116). The engraver provided the pharmacist Duroziez with these thirty-three examples of small-size labels for numerous products on a sheet slightly larger than eight-by-ten inches. Several were for specialties of the pharmacy such as ipecac pills and cucumber pomade, while others, including the "Pilules selon l'ordonn[an]ce" (pills according to the prescription), could be used for individualized orders. The small, round label with an eight-pointed star in its center was to be affixed to the top of the cork when the prescription was dispensed.

116
Labels for
Dr. Michgorius
Dutch, c. 1875
Lithograph
13½ x 8½″ (34.3 x 21.6 cm)
1988-102-10

These long triangular labels for the pharmacy of Dr. Michgorius were affixed to narrow-necked bottles by inserting the smaller end under the cork or cap; they were not pasted on the bottle as they are today. To provide variety, the artist supplied his client with several different illustrations, one of which shows a mortar and pestle resting on an open book inscribed *pharmacie*, with a labeled prescription nearby.

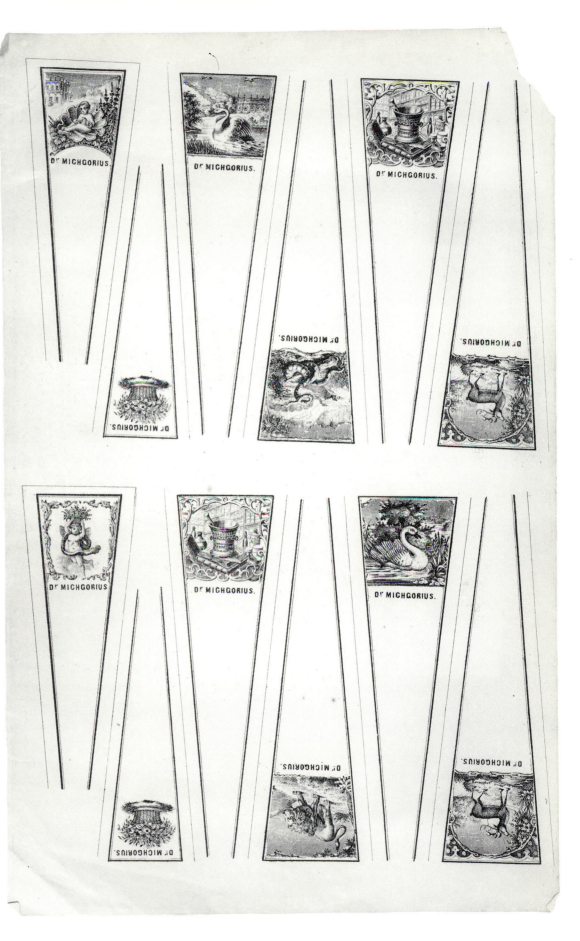

117
Valentine
Quack Doctor
American, c. 1890
Color relief print
9⅝ x 7¹⁄₁₆" (24.5 x 17.9 cm)
(sheet)
1988-102-7

118
Valentine
Dentist
English, 1906
Color lithograph
8¾ x 6¾" (22.2 x 17.2 cm)
1988-104-7

Comic valentines first appeared in Great Britain and North America in the middle of the nineteenth century. They were usually sent anonymously, and were often poorly printed on cheap paper with insulting verses that attacked all trades, professions, and offensive habits such as smoking. Not surprisingly, the health professionals—doctors, pharmacists, dentists, nurses, and their colleagues—came in for their share of abuse, as the examples of the quack doctor and the dentist show.

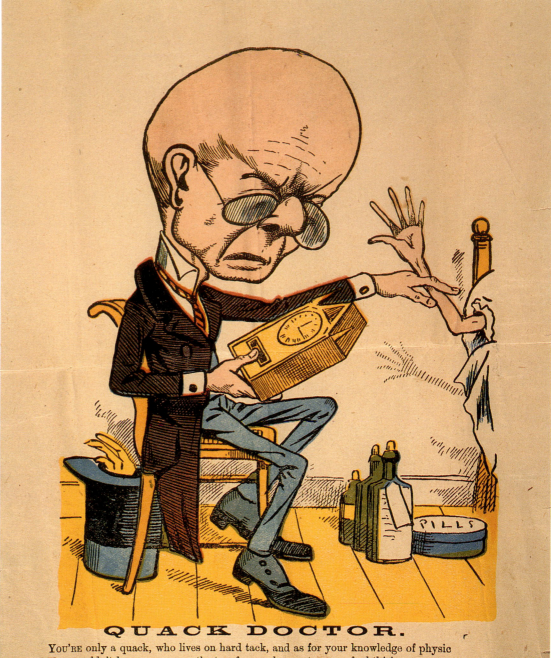

QUACK DOCTOR.

You're only a quack, who lives on hard tack, and as for your knowledge of physic
You wouldn't know a corn on the toe, from a desperate case of phthisic.
Your sugar pill is certain to kill, and as for your lotions and plasters,
They make the sick the worse, empty the purse, and add to our woes and disasters.
The right thing to do, to get rid of you, and end all our troubles and ills,
Is to break the back, of such an old quack, by making him take his own pills.

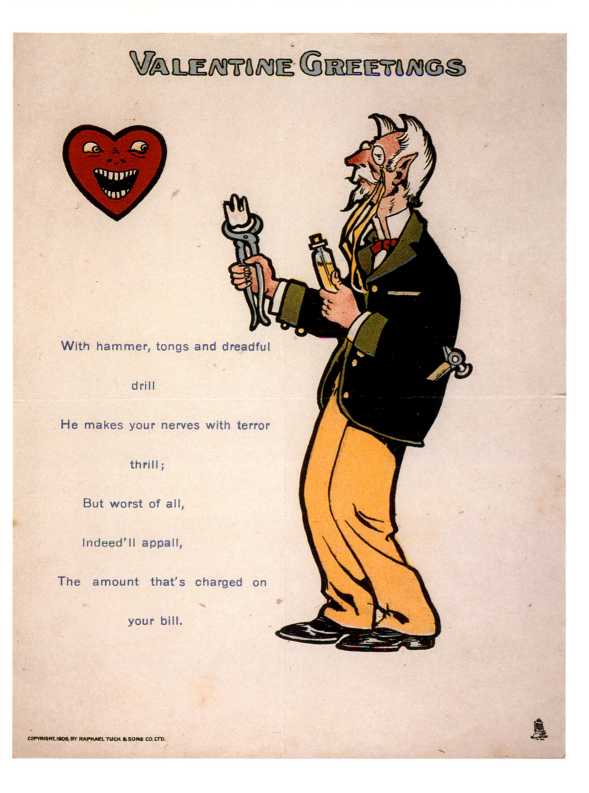

VALENTINE GREETINGS

With hammer, tongs and dreadful

drill

He makes your nerves with terror

thrill;

But worst of all,

Indeed'll appall,

The amount that's charged on

your bill.

119
Sheet Music Cover for
Complaints, or The Ills of Life, with Their Remedies
Alfred Concanen (English, 1835–1886)
1869
Color lithograph
12⅞ x 9⁷⁄₁₆″ (32.7 x 24 cm) (sheet)
1988-102-49

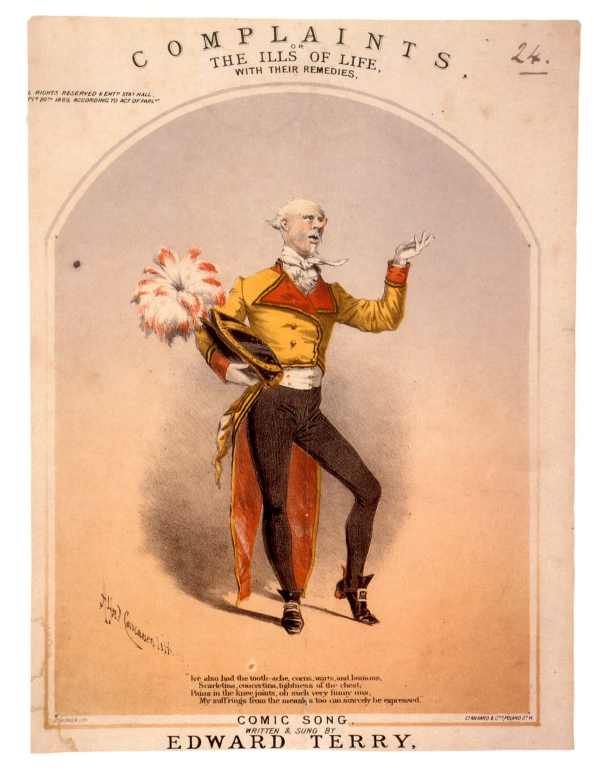

120
Sheet Music Cover for
Poor Pill Garlic
Alfred Concanen (English,
1835–1886)
1877
Color lithograph
13^{15}/$_{16}$ x 10^{3}/$_{16}$" (35.4 x 25.8 cm)
(sheet)
1988-102-50

Instead of choosing images related to the subjects of these two songs, Alfred Concanen drew the entertainers who sang them in their stage costumes. The four-line chorus printed at the bottom of the cover of *Complaints* (no. 119), however, did give prospective purchasers some idea of the contents of the song. As the most popular designer of music covers in England in the late nineteenth century, Concanen produced more than four hundred sheets during his thirty-year career; he also illustrated books and posters.

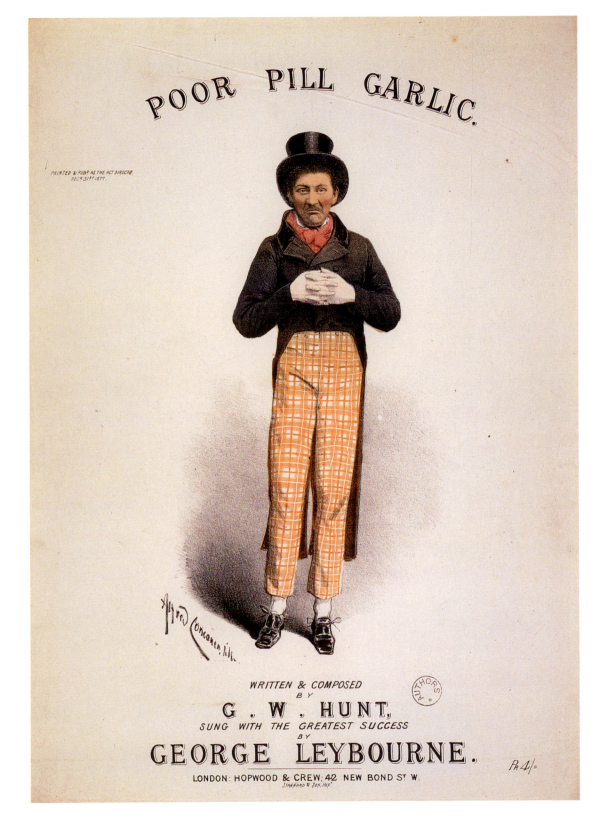

121
Sheet Music Cover for
All Through Obliging a Lady
Alfred Concanen (English,
1835–1886)
c. 1880
Color lithograph
13¹⁵/₁₆ x 9⅝" (35.4 x 24.5 cm)
(sheet)
1988-102-48

Having caught a bad cold "all through obliging a lady," the patient on this song cover has prescribed his own remedies. On his chest he wears an Allcock's Porous Plaster, an unusual rubberized plaster with punched holes that allowed accumulated moisture to escape. The product was developed by Dr. Thomas Allcock in Ossining, New York, and first marketed around 1860. Further, the patient has placed both feet in a solution of Coleman's Mustard and boiling water; he has even bandaged his head to relieve his headache. All of this was the subject of a comic song written and sung by Arthur Lloyd, a well-known music hall performer in Victorian England.

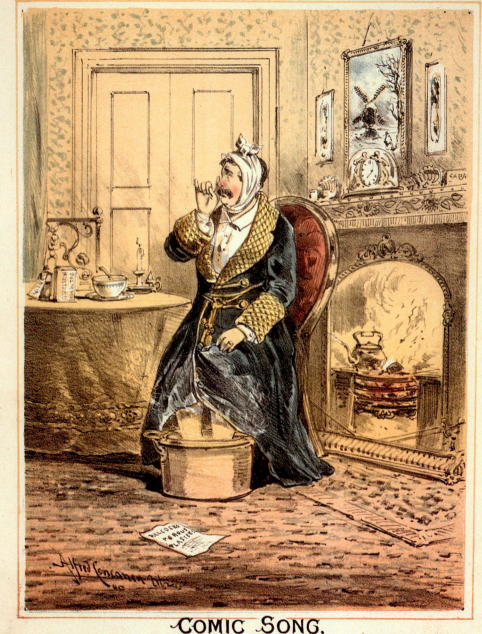

122
Sheet Music Cover for
Amour et rhumatisme
(Love and Rheumatism)
Gustave Donjean (French, n.d.)
c. 1885
Lithograph
13 x 9⁷/₈" (33 x 25 cm) (sheet)
1988-102-72

The comic song *Love and Rheumatism* relates the trials of a young woman who has married a hypochondriacal older man and is forced to be a nurse against her wishes. Despite the smile on her face, she does not recommend her lot to others. Here the "patient" winces as his back is massaged; other requisites for his health — bottles of medicine and a *clyso-pompe*, an enema apparatus popular in nineteenth-century France — are on the night table.

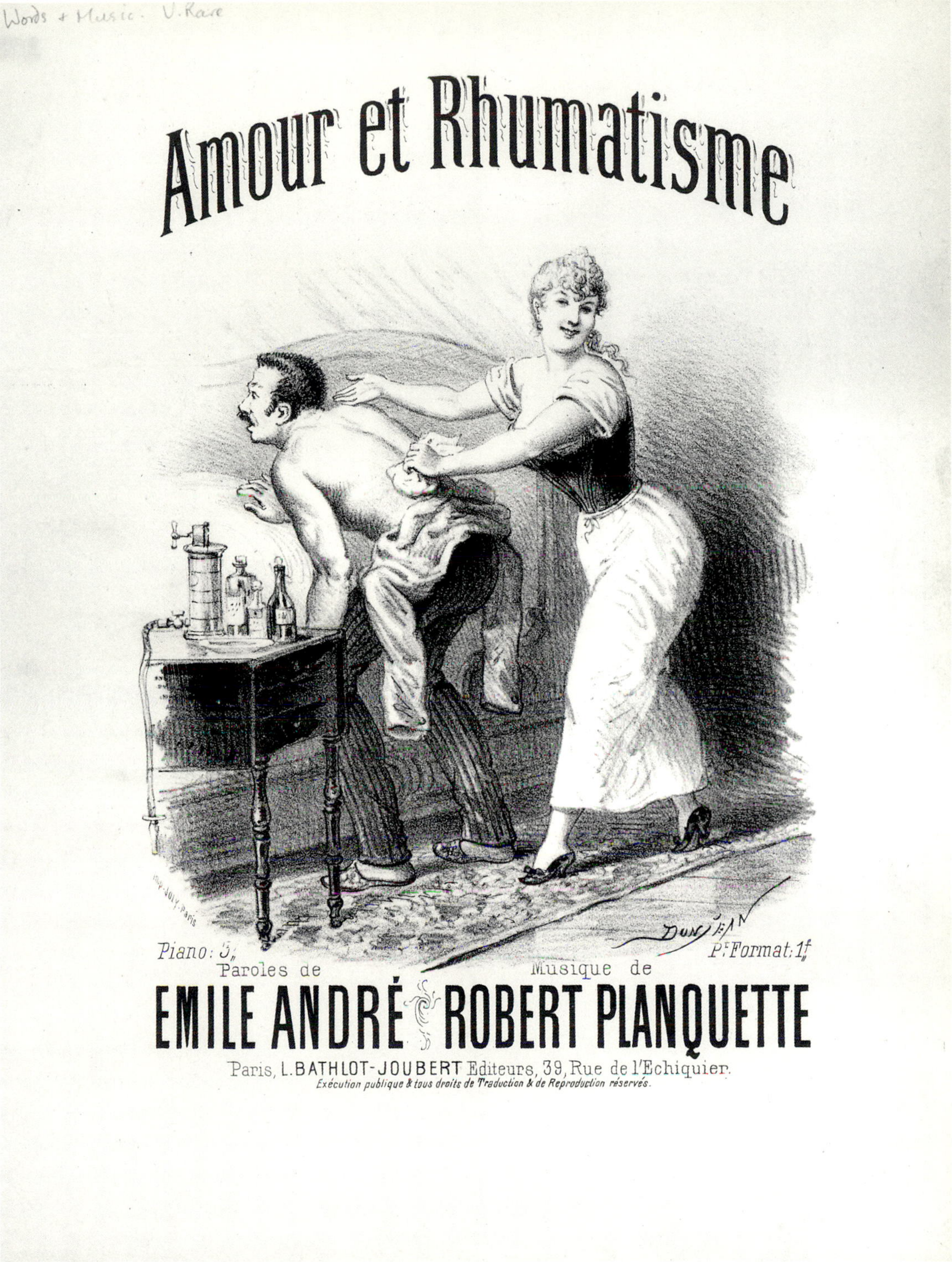

123
Sheet Music Cover for
**The Hypochondriac. Or A Travelling
Doctor's Shop**
H. G. Banks (English, n.d.)
1895
Color lithograph
14 x 10¼" (35.5 x 26 cm) (sheet)
1988-102-40

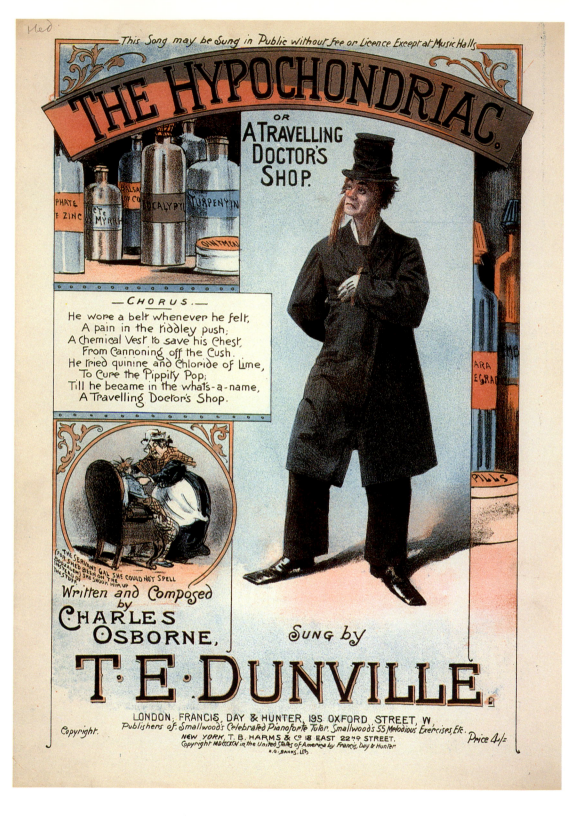

124
Sheet Music Cover for
I'm Studying the Doctor's Orders
H. G. Banks (English, n.d.)
1902
Color lithograph
13½ x 10" (34.3 x 25.4 cm) (sheet)
1988-102-41

The crowded cover for *The Hypochondriac* (no. 123) shows a caricature of the subject of the comic song along with bottles and jars of medicine, a vignette of a servant who stupidly shook the patient instead of the bottle, and even eight lines of the chorus. In *I'm Studying the Doctor's Orders* (no. 124), the illustration is simpler, showing a man carrying a rolled-up mattress, a reference to a line in the chorus of the song: "The doctor said I mustn't leave my bed." Both covers prominently display the name of the singer who performed them on the stage, for entertainers influenced the sales of the sheet music more than words or melodies could.

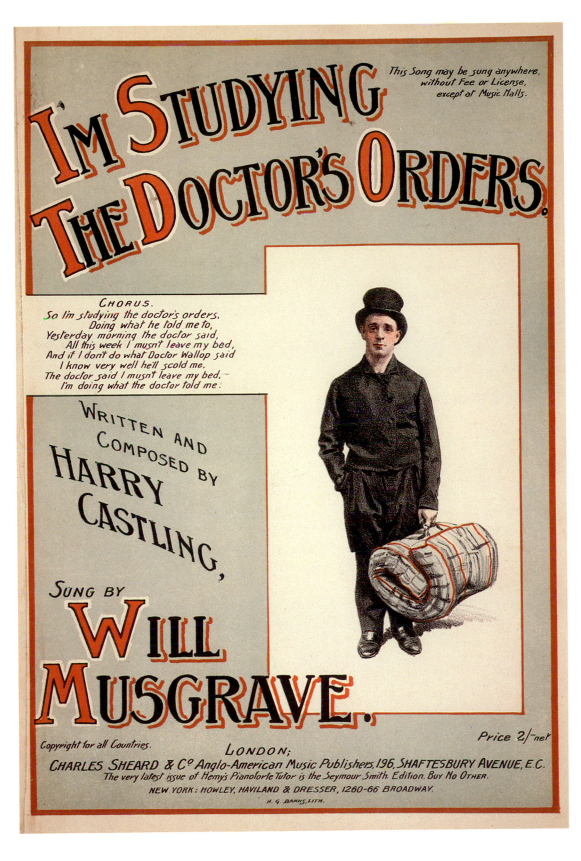

125
Bookplate for
Irene D. Andrews
Michael Fingesten (Austrian,
born 1885)
1939
Soft-ground etching
5¼ x 4⅛" (13.3 x 10.5 cm) (plate)
8¹⁄₁₆ x 6³⁄₁₆" (20.5 x 15.7 cm)
(sheet)
1989-69-11

Fingesten's bookplate for a collection of books on the Dance of Death,
the Bibliotheca Macabrum, includes
vignettes of Death engaged in various activities, such as playing a
violin, being photographed, and
studying his portrait. In the principal
image, Death has spread eleven
cards on a table to tell the future of
wide-eyed young woman.

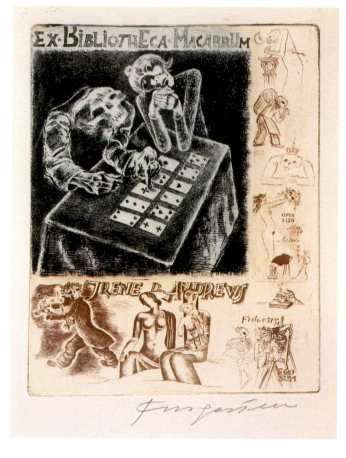

126
Bookplate for
Dr. K. Knauf
Probably German, 1930—40
Woodcut
6½ x 4¼" (16.5 x 10.8 cm)
(image)
7⁹⁄₁₆ x 5³⁄₈" (19.2 x 13.7 cm)
(sheet)
1988-69-8

In what seems to be an even match,
a snarling dragon is attacked by a
child wielding an oversized syringe.
Four lines of verse reflect a positive
attitude toward life:

All in all, in the fight to the finish
You must learn right now
That wounds heal better
When one battles against them.

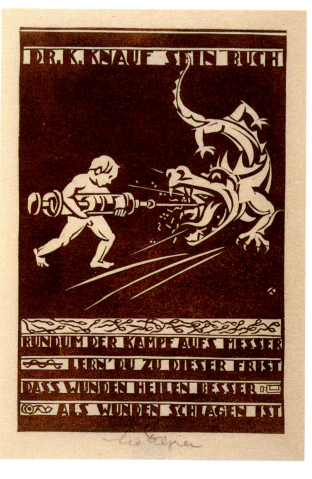

127
Bookplate for
Juan Mercadal
W. Helfenbein (probably
German, n.d.)
1930–40
Etching and aquatint
6³⁄₈ x 3⁷⁄₈" (16.2 x 9.8 cm) (plate)
8¹⁄₄ x 5⁵⁄₈" (21 x 14.3 cm) (sheet)
1989-69-9

A dour chemist, wearing a heavy fur-lined robe, pours from a small bowl into a larger one, and as the liquid reaches the container there is a flash of light. A mortar and pestle and two retorts lie on a table, and there are three bars from *Manfred*, Robert Schumann's 1848–49 composition for soloists, chorus, and orchestra, at the bottom of the plate.

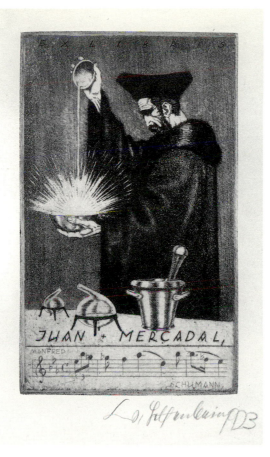

128
Bookplate for
Albert Zeller, Apotheker
Arnold Oechslin (probably
German, n.d.)
1930–40
Etching
6¹⁄₈ x 4³⁄₈" (15.5 x 11.1 cm) (plate)
8¹⁵⁄₁₆ x 5⁵⁄₈" (22.7 x 14.3 cm)
(sheet)
1989-69-10

In fulfilling bookplate commissions, artists often used images of the profession and interests of their patrons. Thus a pharmacy outfitted with rows of drug containers, a scale, and a mortar and pestle is the setting for the bookplate of Albert Zeller, a German apothecary. Zeller's other interests — horse racing, motoring, and sightseeing — are also included in vignettes at the bottom of the composition. As the main image, the artist has drawn an intent pharmacist studying his text, oblivious to the coiling snake at his feet.

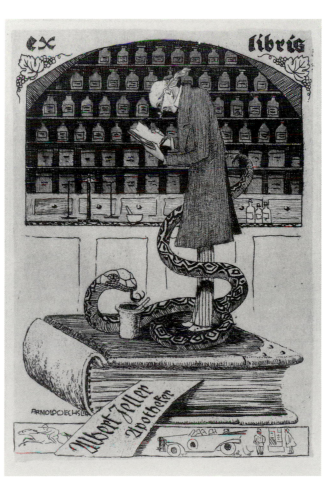

Selected Bibliography

Boyer, Patricia Eckert. *In Sickness and in Health: Medicine and Health Care in 19th-Century French Prints. A Salute to the New Jersey Pharmaceutical Industry.* New Brunswick, 1984. Exhibition, The Jane Voorhees Zimmerli Art Museum, Rutgers, The State University of New Jersey, New Brunswick, June 10—August 19, 1984.

Cowen, David L., and Helfand, William H. *Pharmacy: An Illustrated History.* New York, 1990.

George, M. Dorothy. *English Political Caricature to 1792: A Study of Opinion and Propaganda.* Oxford, 1959.

George, M. Dorothy. *English Political Caricature, 1793–1832: A Study of Opinion and Propaganda.* Oxford, 1959.

Hein, Wolfgang-Hagen. *Die Pharmazie in der Karikatur/Pharmacy in Caricature.* Ingelheim am Rhein, 1964.

Helfand, William H. "Art in the Service of Public Health: The Illustrated Poster." *Caduceus,* vol. 6, no. 2 (Summer 1990), pp. 1–37.

Helfand, William H. *Medicine & Pharmacy in American Political Prints (1765–1870).* Madison, 1978.

Höllander, Eugen. *Die Karikatur und Satire in der Medizin: Mediko-Kunsthistorische Studie.* 2nd ed. Stuttgart, 1921.

Karp, Diane R., et al. *Ars Medica: Art, Medicine, and the Human Condition. Prints, Drawings, and Photographs from the Collection of the Philadelphia Museum of Art.* Philadelphia, 1985. Exhibition, September 22–December 1, 1985.

Lewis, John. *Collecting Printed Ephemera: A Background to Social Habits and Social History, to Eating and Drinking, to Travel and Heritage, and Just for Fun.* London, 1976.

Lewis, John. *Printed Ephemera: The Changing Uses of Type and Letterforms in English and American Printing.* Ipswich, 1962.

Lyons, Albert S., and Petrucelli, R. Joseph, II. *Medicine: An Illustrated History.* New York, 1978.

Mondor, Henri, and Adhémar, Jean. *Doctors & Medicine in the Works of Daumier.* Boston, 1960.

New York State Museum, The State Education Department, Albany. *Medicine & Pharmacy: 100 Years of Poster Art.* October 5, 1981–January 3, 1982. Catalogue by William H. Helfand.

"La Press et l'édition médicale" (entire issue). *Le Courrier graphique,* no. 20 (December 1938).

"La Publicité pharmaceutique" (entire issue). *Le Courrier graphique,* no. 15 (May 1938).

Rickards, Maurice. *Collecting Printed Ephemera.* Oxford, 1988.

Ring, Malvin E. *Dentistry: An Illustrated History.* New York, 1985.

Sturani, Enrico. *Curarsi con le cartoline.* Rome, 1983.

Veth, Cornelis, ed. *Der Arzt in der Karikatur.* Berlin, n.d. [1927].

Weber, A. *Tableau de la caricature médicale depuis les origines jusqu'à nos jours.* Paris, 1936.

Wechsler, Judith. *A Human Comedy: Physiognomy and Caricature in 19th Century Paris.* Chicago, 1982.

Zigrosser, Carl. *Ars Medica: A Collection of Medical Prints by Great Artists of the Past Presented to the Art Museum by Smith, Kline, & French Laboratories.* Philadelphia, 1955. 2nd ed., rev. and enl., Philadelphia, 1959. Published as *Medicine and the Artist,* 3rd ed., rev. and enl., New York, 1970.

Index

Published on the occasion of an exhibition at the Philadelphia Museum of Art, September 21–December 1, 1991

Designed by Phillip Unetic
Edited by Sherry Babbitt
Composition by Southern New England Typographic Service, Hamden, Connecticut
Printed by Princeton Polychrome Press, Princeton, New Jersey

Distributed by the
University of Pennsylvania Press
418 Service Drive
Philadelphia, Pennsylvania
19104-6097

In dimensions, height precedes width.

All works illustrated are in the William H. Helfand Collection of the Philadelphia Museum of Art, unless noted.

Library of Congress Cataloging-in-Publication Data

Helfand, William H.
   The picture of health : images of medicine and pharmacy from the William H. Helfand Collection : commentaries by William H. Helfand; essays by Patricia Eckert Boyer, Judith Wechsler, and Maurice Rickards.
      p.   cm.
   Includes bibliographical references and index.
   ISBN 0-8122-7962-X (University of Pennsylvania Press) : —
ISBN 0-87633-087-1 (paper : Philadelphia Museum of Art) :
   1. Medicine in art—Exhibitions.
2. Pharmacy in art—Exhibitions.
3. Art—Exhibitions. 4. Helfand, William H.—Art collections—Exhibitions. 5. Art—Private collections—Pennsylvania—Philadelphia—Exhibitions. 6. Philadelphia Museum of Art—Exhibitions. I. Boyer, Patricia Eckert. II. Wechsler, Judith, 1940–   .
III. Rickards, Maurice, 1919–   .
IV. Philadelphia Museum of Art.
V. Title.
N8223.H44   1991
769'.4961—dc20   91-19745
                              CIP

Photographic Credits

Joan Broderick: no. 2; Andrew Harkins: nos. 16, 17, 22, 24, 26–29, 31, 33–54, 57, 58, 60–128; Eric Mitchell: nos. 4, 12, 25; Graydon Wood: nos. 1, 3, 5–11, 13–15, 18–21, 23, 30, 32, 55, 56, 59